1D90
£14.95

Practical Gynaecology

Related titles

Contemporary Gynaecology, edited by Geoffrey Chamberlain

Contraception: Science and Practice, edited by Marcus Filshie and John Guillebaud

Dewhurst's Paediatric and Adolescent Gynaecology, 2nd edn, edited by D. K. Edmonds

Labour Ward Manual, by David Liu and Denys Fairweather

Principles of Gynaecology, 4th edn, by T. N. A. Jeffcoate

Principles of Obstetrics, by Bryan M. Hibbard

Handbook of Obstetrics and Gynaecology: A Guide for Housemen and Midwives, by R. S. Ledward

Undergraduate Obstetrics and Gynaecology, 2nd edn, by M. G. R. Hull, Gillian Turner and D. N. Joyce

Practical Gynaecology

David T. Y. Liu MPhil(BioEng), MB, BS, FRCOG
Senior Lecturer/Consultant, Department of Obstetrics and Gynaecology, City Hospital, Queens Medical Centre, Nottingham

Gillian C. L. Lachelin MA, MD, FRCOG
Reader and Honorary Consultant in Obstetrics and Gynaecology, University College and Middlesex School of Medicine, London

Butterworths
London Boston Singapore Sydney Toronto Wellington

PART OF REED INTERNATIONAL P.L.C.

First published 1989

British Library Cataloguing in Publication Data
Liu, D.T.Y. (David Tek-Yung)
Practical gynaecology
1. Gynaecology
I. Title II. Lachelin, Gillian C.L.
618.1

ISBN 0-407-00580-3

Library of Congress Cataloging in Publication Data
Liu, D.T.Y.
Practical gynaecology/David T.Y. Liu, Gillian Lachelin.
p. cm.
Includes bibliographies and index.
ISBN 0-407-00580-3
1. Gynecology. I. Lachelin, Gillian C.L.
[DNLM: 1. Genital Diseases, Female. WP 140 L783p]
RG101.L526 1989
618.1--dc19
DNLM/DLC 88-7451
CIP

Typeset by The Alden Press Oxford London and Northampton
Printed in Great Britain at the University Press, Cambridge

Preface

There are many textbooks on gynaecology but few offer practical assistance in the management of patients as they present in the clinic or surgery. The aim of this book is to provide a practical reference manual which gives clear guidance on the appropriate management of patients presenting with gynaecological problems.

Acknowledgements

We are indebted to many past teachers and authors and also to several contemporary colleagues including Professor H.A. Brant, Dr M. Katz, Dr V. Little, Dr G.L. Ridgway, Dr P.F. Serhal, Mr A.C. Silverstone, Dr Peter Twining and Dr P.J.M. Watney for their helpful criticisms and useful advice in the preparation of this book. We appreciate the assistance given to us by Mr G. Gilbert (medical photographer) and Sisters P. Thwaites and C. Preston and also thank Mr Philip Ball for drawing the diagrams. We are also very grateful to Miss G. Gregory and Mrs L. Knight-Smith for their invaluable secretarial assistance.

To all those who care for and care about women

Contents

Chapter 1

The gynaecological patient

Gynaecological patients require a particularly sensitive and sympathetic approach. It is often not easy for a woman to consult a doctor with gynaecological symptoms about which she may be embarrassed. She may present with one symptom when her main concern is another gynaecological problem which she is reluctant to discuss until she has assessed the attitude of the doctor. She will want to determine whether she will get a sympathetic reception or not.

Thus, a teenager may complain of vaginal discharge when she wants to discuss contraception or an older woman may complain of lower abdominal pain when her problems are psychosexual. The referral letter may not be informative as to the reason for the patient's visit.

Role of the doctor

- The doctor may be called upon to give medical advice, to be a sympathetic listener, a marriage guidance counseller, a psychosexual adviser or a friend and confidant. The patient has presented for a reason, be it for advice, reassurance or sympathetic support and it is very important to determine her real reason for attending.
- A young doctor may find it difficult to interpret the signals, and assistance from a senior colleague is essential when a woman presents for the first time and often when she returns for a follow-up appointment. It can be difficult to differentiate pyschosomatic symptoms from those with a physical basis.
- The doctor must be a good listener but must also be able to direct the consultation by asking appropriate questions. Different patients will respond best to different approaches and the doctor must adjust to the needs of the patient.
- It is important to appreciate the special needs and concerns of different ethnic and religious groups. Whenever possible, the patient's wishes should be respected and incorporated into the plan of management.
- The patient seeking specialist advice is in a vulnerable position. Gynaecologists can advise but must not impose their views on patients without consideration of alternative lines of management.
- Surgery should not be used as a substitute for proper counselling. Many surgical procedures such as hysterectomy and sterilization can have a substantial psychological impact and the advantages and disadvantages must be very carefully considered before arranging such forms of treatment.
- It must be accepted by the patient and the doctor that even the best efforts may not produce the result that the patient desires. The patient must be kept honestly informed at each stage of management and her trust and respect will then be maintained.

History

The aim of good history taking is to determine the relevant facts and at the same time to listen with a 'third ear' for problems which the patient does not mention overtly.

- The gynaecological patient can range in age from a child to an elderly woman. Rapport is best established by a friendly and courteous attitude appropriate to the age and type of patient.
- Gynaecological management is usually dependent on the history and careful history taking is very important. A diagnosis of, for example, amenorrhoea, intermenstrual bleeding or menorrhagia is based on the history and it is important to obtain information that is as accurate as possible.
- The timing of the onset of the symptoms may be relevant, for example, amenorrhoea that began after changing occupation or urge incontinence that started following the death of a partner.
- An obstetric, gynaecological, medical and surgical past history as well as a family and social history are an integral part of gynaecological history taking. Detailed gynaecological questioning is often best left until after a general history has been taken and the patient's confidence has been gained.
- Many questions are necessarily of a personal nature and can cause embarrassment. The doctor must choose the right time to ask such questions – when rapport has been established – and should ask them in a matter-of-fact way which does not cause embarrassment. This is particularly true when there is a psychosexual or subfertility problem.
- It is often appropriate to involve the partner, particularly when the problem is subfertility or psychosexual, but also in the management of problems such as menorrhagia. The social situation and the degree of support available can then be more adequately assessed and the partner can often be usefully involved in the decision-making process.
- It is very important to make an accurate record of the history, examination, investigations and advice given both from the point of view of present and future management and for medicolegal reasons.

Examination

- Patients normally expect to be examined when they attend with a gynaecological problem but, in order to obtain maximum relaxation and information, it is important to establish good rapport with the patient before attempting to examine her.
- Whether the doctor is male or female it is preferable for the examination to be carried out in the presence of a third person, for example, a nurse, another doctor or a student. A child will usually be more relaxed when her mother is present but an adolescent may be more comfortable in her mother's absence.
- Modesty is important at all ages and the examination should be carried out discreetly and without interruption, with a maximum of two observers who are present with the patient's consent.

- *A general examination* (including blood pressure estimation) is carried out with particular regard to general health and to evidence of anaemia and to endocrine function. An examination of the breasts should always be performed. This provides an opportunity to exclude any abnormalities and to advise the woman to examine her breasts every month (in the follicular phase of the cycle if she is menstruating).
- *An abdominal examintion* is performed checking for any abnormality and paying particular attention to the patient's reaction to the examination.
- *A vaginal examination* is performed in the dorsal or left lateral position. It is preceded by inspection of the vulva. Speculum examination of the cervix and vagina is usually undertaken next but this may be preceded by bimanual examination.
- *Speculum examination* is usually performed using a bivalve speculum (Figure 1.1). It is very important to explain to the patient what is going to happen. Gloves are put on and a speculum of appropriate size is selected and lubricated and gently inserted into the vagina in the anteroposterior diameter with the blades closed. The handles

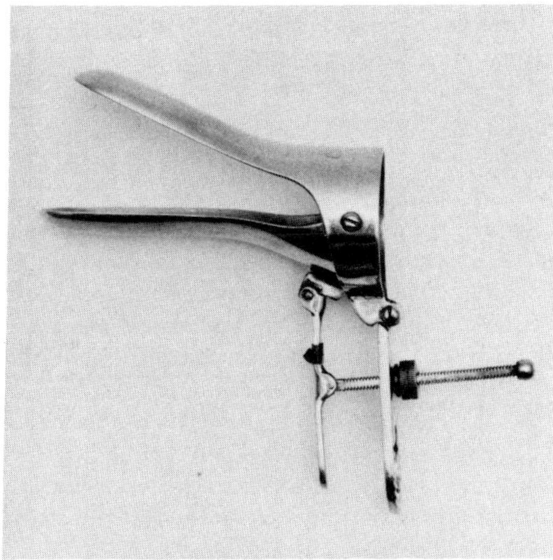

Figure 1.1 Cusco's speculum.

of the speculum are rotated upwards or downwards through 90° during insertion, which should be gentle but positive, and the blades are then opened to expose the cervix which is inspected (Figure 1.2). A cervical smear (see Chapter 18) and swabs are taken if indicated. The vagina is then inspected and swabs taken if indicated. The speculum is gently withdrawn in the closed position taking great care not to pinch the patient.

- *A Sims speculum* (Figures 1.3 and 1.4) is used with the patient in the left lateral position, to inspect the walls of the vagina and to examine for prolapse.
- *Bimanual examination* is usually performed in the dorsal position. The lubricated gloved second and third fingers (or just the second finger if appropriate) of the right hand are introduced into the vagina and the left hand is placed on the lower

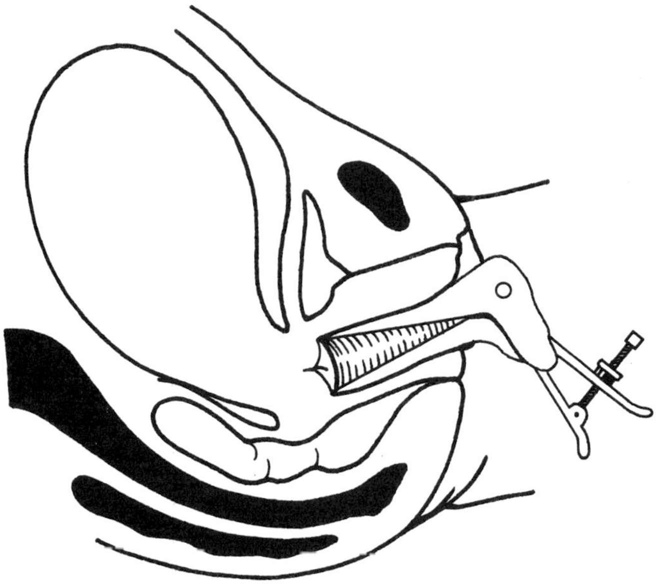

Figure 1.2 Cusco's speculum *in situ.* Handles may be rotated down-wards (as shown) or upwards depending on type of examination couch. (After *Labour Ward Manual,* D.T.Y. Liu and D.V.I. Fairweather, p. 9, 1985, Butterworths).

abdomen. The fingers of the right hand examine the cervix, feeling its consistency and its direction to determine whether the uterus is anteverted or retroverted. The body of the uterus is anteverted if necessary by backward pressure on the cervix and is then felt between the fingers in the vagina and the abdominal hand. After assessment of the position, size, shape, consistency and mobility of the uterus the fingers are then moved laterally first to feel the right and then the left appendages with the help of the abdominal hand. In a slim, relaxed woman it may be possible to feel a normal ovary – particularly on the right side; the ovary is normally tender and should not be pressed too hard. Any masses, thickening or tenderness should be noted as well as any discomfort on moving the cervix (cervical excitation pain).

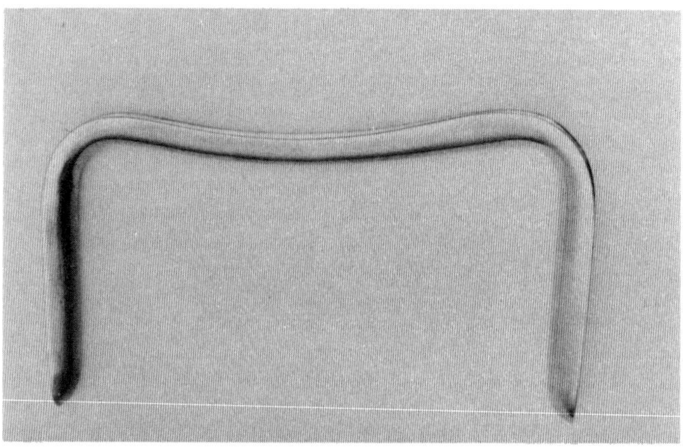

Figure 1.3 Sims speculum.

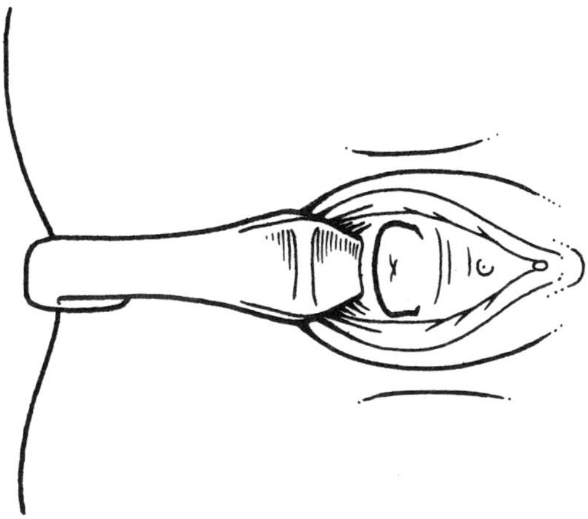

Figure 1.4 Sims speculum *in situ.* (After *Labour Ward Manual,* D.T.Y. Liu and D.V.I. Fairweather, p. 9, 1985, Butterworths).

- It is important to avoid contact with the sensitive clitoris during speculum and bimanual examination.
- Vaginal examination may not always be possible or permitted. A rectal examination may be acceptable and may provide adequate information. General anaesthesia may sometimes be required for adequate examination.

Investigations

- It is important, as in all branches of medicine, neither to under-investigate nor to over-investigate, and to understand the value and limitations of each test.
- An attempt should be made to find out the results of tests that have been adequately performed elsewhere, so that the expense and inconvenience of unnecessary repetition can be avoided.
- The patient can often contribute to her own management by completing, for example, a basal body temperature chart or a menstrual and symptom diary.
- A programme of management should be delineated at the first visit and return visits should be arranged according to this programme and not haphazardly.

Surgical treatment

- If surgery is required, the need for it should be clearly explained. A date should be given, if possible, and the patient should be told where and when to come and what will happen when she is admitted, when she is likely to have the operation (morning or afternoon), what it entails and how long she will be in hospital. Possible after-effects must be discussed and she must be told whether she will need to be off work and if so for how long and what provision, if any, should be made for convalescence. The more that she understands about what is likely to happen the less anxious she will be.

- Some operations should be planned for a specific time in the cycle. Thus, tubal surgery and myomectomy are usually performed in the follicular phase and laparoscopy for investigation of infertility is usually performed in the luteal phase.
- Outpatient investigations such as full blood count and other tests that may be indicated (such as a sickle test, blood grouping, hepatitis screening etc.) should be arranged.
- If the patient is on medication, this should be reviewed and appropriate changes considered in consultation with her physician or general practitioner if necessary.

Preoperative assessment

- There will normally be an interval of days or months before the patient is admitted for surgery.
- The history and indications for surgery must be reviewed to determine whether surgery is still required.
- The date of the last menstrual period must be established and *the possibility of unexpected pregnancy must be excluded.*
- Confirm that the patient is medically fit for the procedure and enquire about any medications she is or has been taking.
- Rediscuss the operation and its possible after-effects. Listen to any concerns the patient may have and reassure her appropriately.
- Obtain signed consent for the procedure that is to be undertaken using the appropriate consent form. (A special form is used for sterilization.)
- Normally the patient will be seen by the anaesthetist who will prescribe premedication, but if not the operating list should be discussed with the anaesthetist and appropriate premedication prescribed as well as any extra medication that may be indicated in particular circumstances, for example, antibiotic or anticoagulant cover, or a prostaglandin pessary prior to termination of pregnancy.
- The patient must have nil by mouth for at least 4–6 hours before surgery.
- The bowel and bladder should preferably be empty before the patient is premedicated.

Postoperative management

- Ensure that the patient is round from the anaesthetic before she returns to the ward.
- Maintain a pulse and blood pressure chart for several hours – the length of time depends on the nature of the operation.
- Monitor any blood loss.
- Provide adequate analgesia.
- Subsequent management will depend on the nature of the operation – see appropriate chapter.
- Following laparotomy, the intravenous infusion should be continued until observa-

tions are stable and bowel sounds are present. If ileus supervenes intravenous hydration must be maintained.

- Urinary retention is common following gynaecological surgery and must be watched out for. All patients who have had major surgery should be on an input–output chart for at least 24 hours.
- A slight pyrexia of around 38°C is common following laparotomy but this usually settles in 24–48 hours. Any subsequent fever must be thoroughly investigated to determine the source, e.g. urinary tract infection, haematoma formation, wound infection, chest infection or thrombosis.
- Early mobilization should be encouraged with physiotherapy as necessary.
- Explain to the patient what was found at the time of surgery, and what was done and what the consequences are for the future. If there was preoperative concern about malignancy, reassure the patient or explain to her what the situation is as appropriate. Reassure all patients when the histology comes back, if it is benign, as many will be concerned about the possibility of malignancy even if they have not expressed their fears.
- If some unexpected problem arises during surgery with, for example, damage to another structure, it is very important that the surgeon explains to the patient what the problem was and what any possible consequences are. Full and open explanation and reassurance at this stage is the best approach.

Discharge from hospital

- Ensure that the patient is fit to go home and that she understands the nature of the surgery performed and the need for any special precautions.
- Make sure that she has a certificate if necessary and that she knows when it will be appropriate for her to return to work.
- Provide her with any necessary medication and a follow-up appointment if required.
- Give her a brief summary to take home with her in case any problems arise and send a copy to the general practitioner or communicate by telephone if necessary.

Discharge from the clinic

It is important to know when to discharge a patient from the clinic. She should be discharged if her problem is resolved or if she is on satisfactory maintenance therapy, or if no further useful treatment is available from the clinic which she is attending. In the latter case, further referral may be appropriate, for example in unexplained infertility or in a patient with psychosexual problems.

Summary

In summary, the management of the gynaecological patient should be sensitive, logical and appropriate and the patient should be kept informed at every stage.

Chapter 2

Anatomy of the female genital tract

Vulva (Figure 2.1)

Mons pubis

- Fatty tissue over symphysis pubis.
- Overlying skin contains sebaceous and sweat glands and is covered with coarse pubic hair.

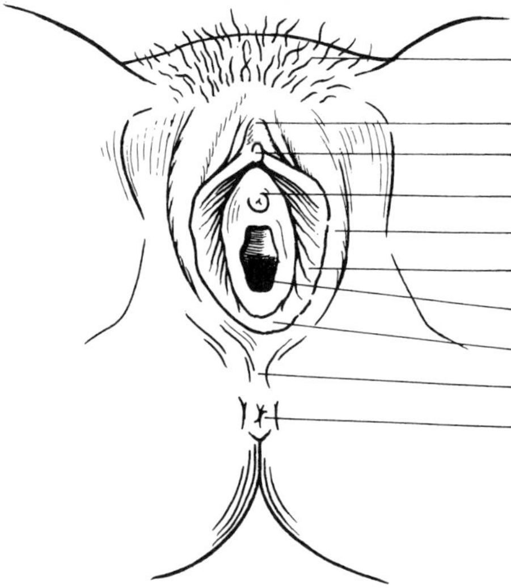

Figure 2.1 Anatomy of the vulva.

Labia majora

- Folds of fatty tissue continuous with mons pubis anteriorly.
- Covered with skin containing hair follicles (on lateral surfaces) and sebaceous and sweat glands.
- Homologous with scrotum – formed from genital swellings.

Labia minora

- Thin folds of skin between labia majora.
- Anteriorly form prepuce and frenulum of clitoris.
- Contain sebaceous and sweat glands but no hair follicles.

- More prominent than labia majora in children and postmenopausally.
- Homologous with phallic portion of male urethra – formed from genital folds.

Clitoris

- Consists of crura (attached to pubic rami), body and very sensitive glans.
- Crura and body are composed of erectile tissue.
- Homologous with penis – formed from genital tubercle.

Vestibule

- Bounded by labia minora and fourchette.
- Urethra, vagina and Bartholin's glands open onto it.

Hymen

- Thin membrane at junction of vestibule and vagina covered with stratified squamous epithelium.
- Usually perforate, sometimes with more than one aperture.
- Hymenal remnants represented by carunculae myrtiformes.

Bartholin's glands

- Lie posterolateral to vaginal orifice at 5 and 7 o'clock; acini lined by columnar epithelium.
- Produce colourless mucoid secretion which acts as lubricant in response to sexual arousal.
- Ducts approximately 2 cm long open into introitus below hymen. Lined by transitional epithelium.
- Neither glands nor ducts normally palpable or visible.

Perineal body

- Lies between lower third of vagina and anal canal.
- Point of insertion of perineal muscles (bulbospongiosus, pubococcygeus, and superficial and deep transverse perineal muscles), as well as posterior border of urogenital diaphragm and anterior fibres of sphincter ani.

Blood supply of vulva

- Internal pudendal artery and anteriorly superficial external pudendal artery.
- Venous drainage accompanies arterial supply, also via vesical and vaginal plexuses.

Lymphatic drainage of vulva

- To superficial inguinal nodes and deep inguinal, femoral and external iliac nodes.

Vagina

- Fibromuscular distensible tube extending from vestibule to cervix.
- Anterior and posterior walls are in apposition.
- Runs upwards and backwards at angle of approximately 45° to horizontal.
- Anterior wall is shorter than posterior wall which is about 10 cm long.
- Closely related anteriorly to urethra and base of bladder.
- Closely related posteriorly to perineal body, rectum and pouch of Douglas (Figure 2.2).

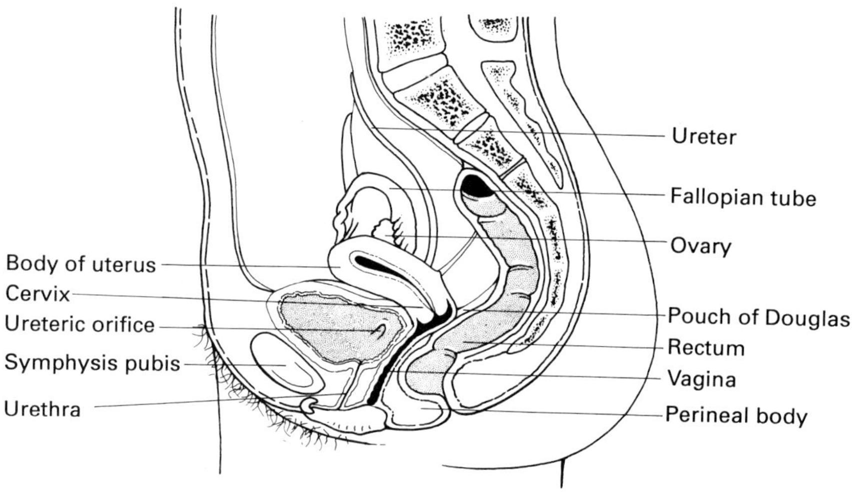

Figure 2.2 Sagittal section through pelvis.

- Lined by stratified squamous epithelium which is in transverse folds or rugae; it has no glands.
- Under oestrogen stimulation, epithelium produces glycogen from which lactic acid is formed by action of Döderlein's bacilli, following desquamation.
- Normal pH in reproductive life is approximately 4.5; rises during menstruation. Higher in childhood and postmenopausally because of lower oestrogen levels.

Embryology of vagina

- Formed from vaginal plate (which is composed of urogenital sinus epithelium and paramesonephric duct tissue).
- Initially solid, but normally canalization occurs at 16–18 weeks' intrauterine life forming vaginal lumen.

Blood supply of vagina

- Vaginal artery, branches of uterine artery, internal pudendal artery, and middle and inferior rectal arteries.
- Venous drainage by vaginal plexus to internal iliac veins.

Lymphatic drainage of vagina

- The drainage from the lower vagina is the same as the vulva; the drainage from the upper vagina is the same as the cervix.

Uterus

- Composed of body (corpus) and cervix (neck).
- In reproductive age group, about 8–10 cm long, 5–6 cm wide at widest point and 2.5–3 cm from front to back.
- In children much smaller and cervix is longer than body.
- In postmenopausal women uterus shrinks and cervix may become flush with vaginal vault.
- Anteverted in about 80% of women. Maintained in anteversion by its weight, the round ligaments (which are inserted at uterine cornua and run in the broad ligaments to the inguinal canals) and the uterosacral ligaments (which run from the supravaginal cervix to the periosteum of the sacrum and keep the cervix pulled back).
- Main ligamentary supports of the uterus are the transverse cervical (cardinal) ligaments which fan out from the supravaginal cervix to the pelvic wall.
- Ureters lie only 1–2 cm lateral to supravaginal cervix passing just below the uterine arteries.

Body of uterus

- Globular muscular organ flattened from front to back with triangular (endometrial) cavity whose front and back walls are in apposition.
- Covered by intimately adherent peritoneum except at sides between leaves of broad ligaments and on lower anterior wall which is covered by loosely attached peritoneum of uterovesical pouch.
- Myometrium (1–1.5 cm thick) consists of bundles of smooth muscle arranged in three layers, the middle layer being the thickest.
- Endometrium consists of basal layer not shed at time of menstruation and superficial layers which undergo changes during the menstrual cycle and which are shed at the time of menstruation (see Chapter 3).

Cervix

- Cylindrical, about 2.5 cm long, composed of fibromuscular and collagenous tissue.
- Half projects into vagina (vaginal cervix) and half lies above it (supravaginal cervix).
- Cervical canal runs from internal to external os.
- External os is small and circular in nulliparous women, but is often a transverse slit in parous women.
- Endocervix is lined by folds of columnar epithelium which form anterior and posterior columns with circumferentially radiating folds – the so-called arbor vitae.
- Branched glands penetrate deeply into fibromuscular stroma.
- Secretion from glands increases under oestrogen stimulation to form mucus suitable for penetration by sperms around time of ovulation.

Embryology of uterus and cervix

- Formed by fusion and canalization of paramesonephric (müllerian) ducts.
- Abnormalities of development, of fusion and of canalization can occur resulting in unicornuate uterus, bicornuate uterus, uterine septum, rudimentary horn etc. (Figure 2.3).

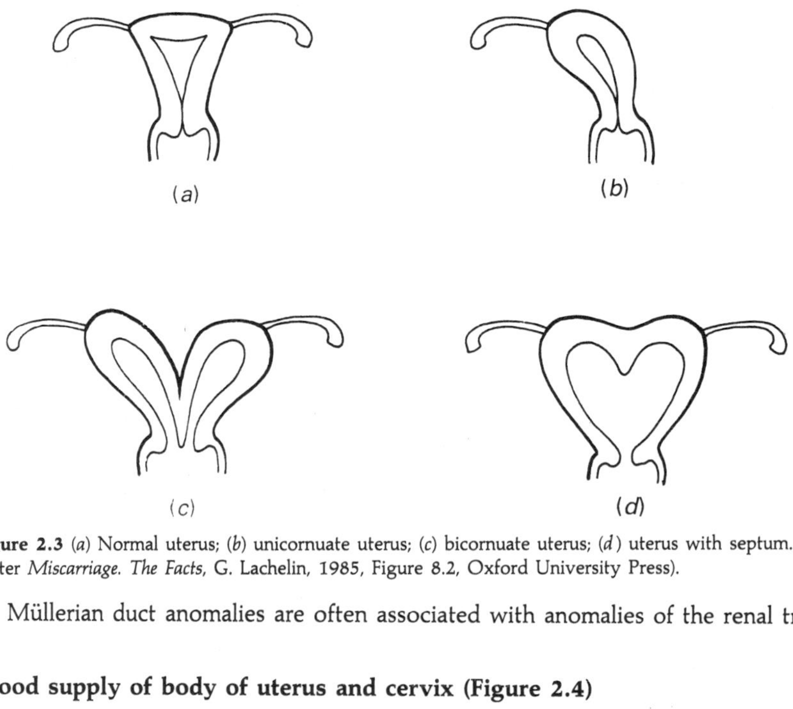

Figure 2.3 (*a*) Normal uterus; (*b*) unicornuate uterus; (*c*) bicornuate uterus; (*d*) uterus with septum. (After *Miscarriage. The Facts*, G. Lachelin, 1985, Figure 8.2, Oxford University Press).

- Müllerian duct anomalies are often associated with anomalies of the renal tract.

Blood supply of body of uterus and cervix (Figure 2.4)

- From uterine (branch of internal iliac) and ovarian (arise directly from the aorta) arteries.

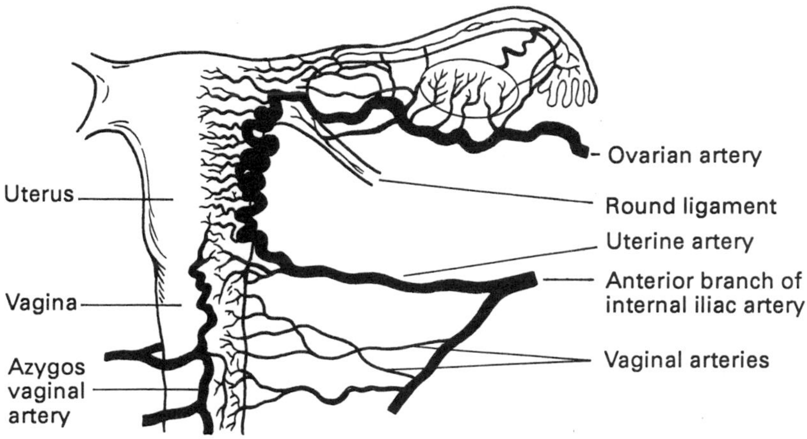

Figure 2.4 Blood supply of genital tract.

- Venous drainage is via uterine and ovarian veins.

Lymphatic drainage of body of uterus and cervix (Figure 2.5)

- From upper part of uterus, drainage is to para-aortic nodes (via lymphatics accompanying ovarian vessels) and occasionally to superficial and deep inguinal nodes via lymphatics in the round ligaments.
- From lower part of the uterus and cervix, drainage is mainly to paracervical, parametrial, internal and external iliac nodes and the obturator node.

Fallopian tubes

- Fibromuscular oviducts about 10 cm long running in upper margin of broad ligaments from cornua of uterus to ovaries.
- Divided into four parts:
  1. Interstitial portion <1 mm internal diameter runs through muscular wall of uterine cornu.
  2. Isthmus <1 mm internal diameter, 2–3 mm external diameter and 2–3 cm long runs from the cornu to the ampulla.
  3. Ampulla, about 6 mm external diameter and 5–6 cm long, runs from isthmus to infundibulum.
  4. Infundibulum – dilated outer end of tube which ends in finger-like fimbriae.
- The tubes are lined by mucous membrane, most elaborately plicated in ampulla and infundibulum and composed of columnar epithelial cells many of which are ciliated.

Embryology of fallopian tubes

- Develop from the upper part of müllerian ducts.

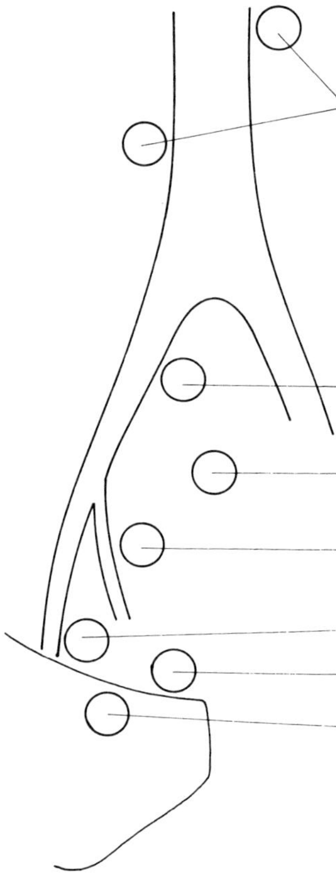

Figure 2.5 Schematic representation of lymph nodes draining the genital tract.

Ovaries

- White structures with irregular surface measuring about 3 × 2 × 1.5 cm.
- Suspended from uterine cornua by ovarian ligaments and attached to back of broad ligaments by mesovarium.
- Composed of stroma and follicles (primordial, maturing, degenerating and atretic).

Embryology of ovaries

- Formed from coelomic epithelium of the genital ridge, the underlying mesoderm and germ cells from beneath the epithelium of the yolk sac.
- By 20 weeks of intrauterine life, there are several million germ cells in the ovary but only 1–2 million are present at term and only a few hundred thousand by the time of the menarche. No new germ cells are produced after birth. The situation is therefore quite different from that in the male where spermatogenesis normally occurs throughout adult life.

Blood supply of ovaries

- Ovarian arteries and, to a lesser extent, uterine arteries.
- Venous drainage is by ovarian veins, uterine veins and broad ligament plexuses.

Lymphatic drainage of ovaries

- To para-aortic nodes.

Chapter 3

Physiology of the menstrual cycle

The menstrual cycle is controlled by a complex hormonal interplay involving the hypothalamus, pituitary, ovaries and uterus. An abnormality at any of these levels can result in disruption of the normal menstrual cycle.

Luteinizing hormone-releasing hormone (LHRH) produced by the hypothalamus stimulates production and release of follicle stimulating hormone (FSH) and luteinizing hormone (LH) by the pituitary. These gonadotrophins stimulate the ovary to produce androgens, oestrogens and progesterone which have feedback effects on the hypothalamus and pituitary and thus modulate the production and release of gonadotrophins.

Hormones

- *LHRH* (luteinizing hormone-releasing hormone) is a decapeptide produced by the hypothalamus. It is produced in pulsatile fashion and has a very short half-life. Synthetic LHRH can be used in the treatment of some forms of anovulation and is given in pulses, usually every 90 minutes, using an infusion pump. Various analogues with much longer half-lives have been produced and are currently mainly used to achieve ovarian suppression.
- *FSH* and *LH* are glycoproteins with a molecular weight of about 30 000. They each consist of an α- and a β-subunit; the α-subunit of all the pituitary glycoproteins and of human chorionic gonadotrophin (HCG) is similar but the β-subunits differ. The similarity of the α-subunits explains the considerable cross-reaction between LH and HCG in routine radioimmunoassays; the βHCG-subunit assay has been developed to overcome this problem. The fluctuations in peripheral FSH and LH levels during the menstrual cycle are shown diagrammatically in Figure 3.1.
- *FSH* stimulates ovarian follicular development and oestrogen production.
- *LH* stimulates androgen production; in addition the midcycle LH surge is responsible for inducing ovulation from a ripe follicle and for the formation of the corpus luteum. Because of the structural similarity between the α-subunits of LH and HCG, HCG (5000–10 000 units) can be used therapeutically to mimic the LH surge.
- *Oestrogens* – these are C_{18} steroids produced from androgen precursors (Figure 3.2). Oestradiol is produced by the developing follicle and the corpus luteum and by peripheral conversion from androgens and oestrone. Oestrone is produced by peripheral conversion from androstenedione and also by the ovary. Rising oestradiol levels in the early follicular phase stimulate pituitary LH and FSH production and finally cause the LH surge (see Figure 3.1). Oestrogen production is continued by the corpus luteum but decreases as the corpus luteum degenerates if pregnancy does not occur. Implantation is followed by HCG production by the developing conceptus and this maintains the corpus luteum and stimulates continued ovarian steroid production in early pregnancy.

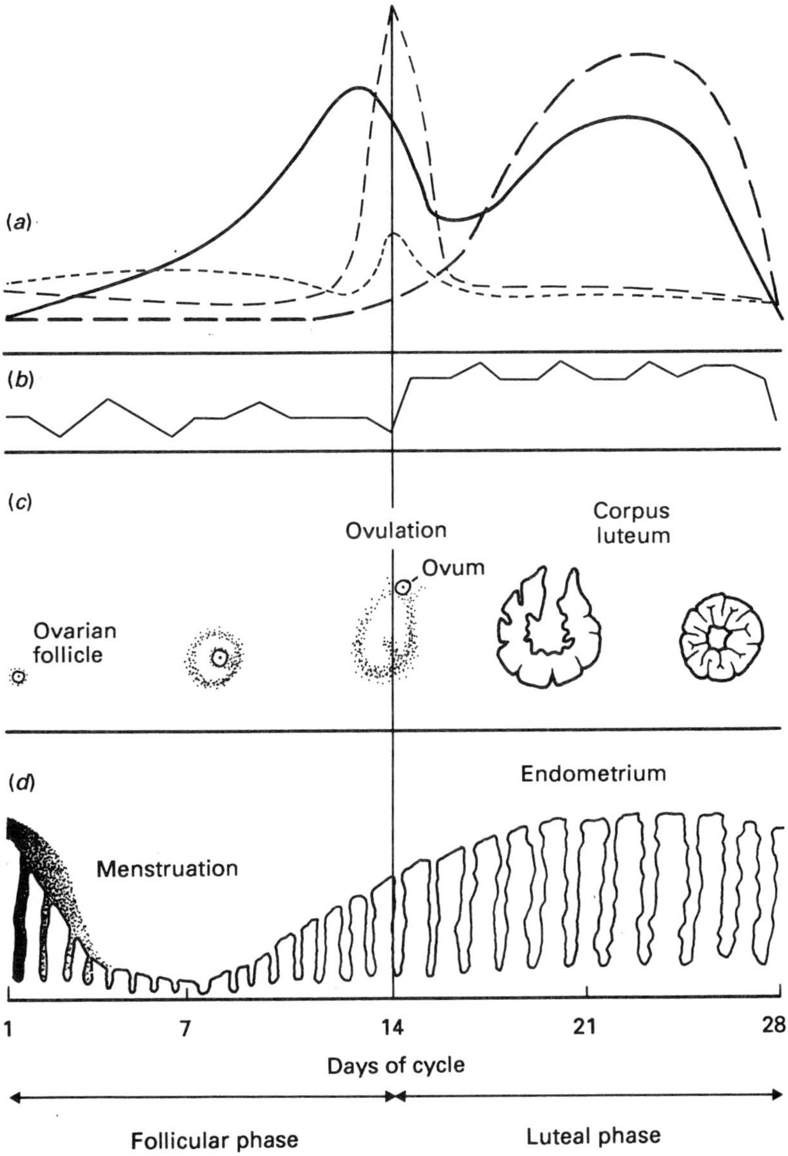

Figure 3.1 The menstrual cycle. (*a*) Hormonal events: ---- FSH; — — — LH; ——— oestradiol; — — progesterone. (*b*) Body temperature; (*c*) ovarian events; (*d*) uterine events. (From *Miscarriage. The Facts*, G. Lachelin, 1985, Figure 3.1, Oxford University Press, by permission).

- *Androgens* are C_{19} steroids secreted by the ovaries and adrenal cortex. The main androgens secreted by the ovaries are androstenedione and testosterone which act as precursors for oestrogen production both in the ovary and in the periphery. The main androgen secreted by the adrenal cortex is dehydroepiandrosterone (Figure 3.2).

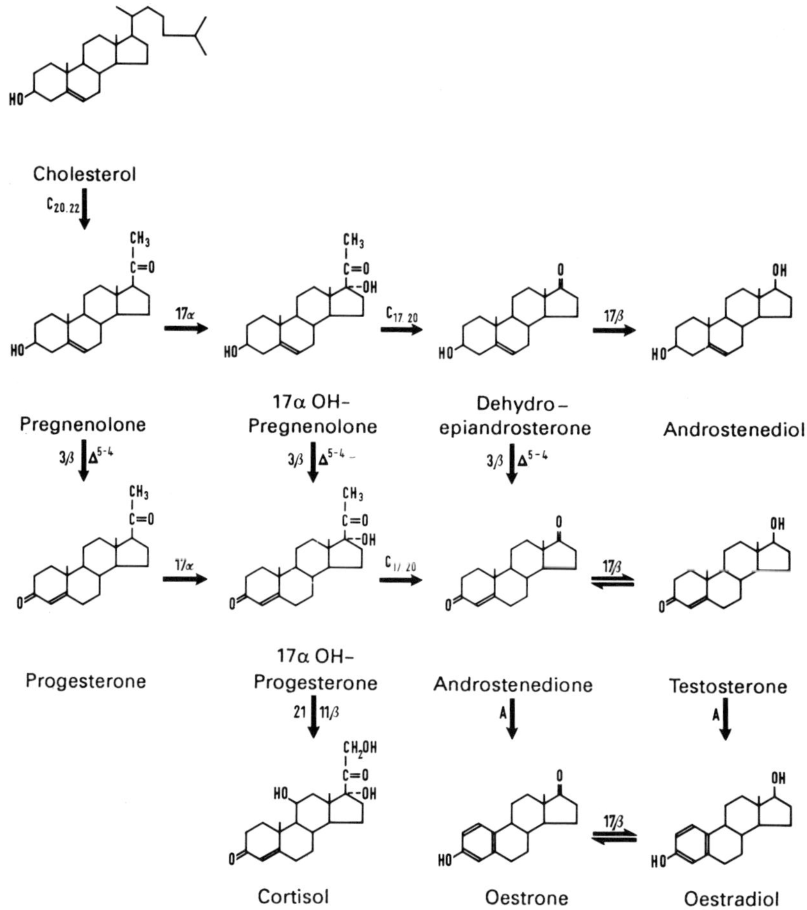

Figure 3.2 Steroid pathways: $C_{20.22}$ = $C_{20,22}$ desmolase: 3 $\beta\Delta^{5-4}$ = Δ^{5-4}-3βOH dehydrogenase and $\Delta^5$4-isomerase; 17α = 17α-hydroxylase; 17β = 17β-reductase; 21 = 21-hydroxylase; 11β = 11β-hydroxylase; $C_{17.20}$ = $C_{17.20}$ desmolase; A = aromatase.

- *Progesterone* is a C_{21} steroid secreted mainly by the corpus luteum. It causes changes in the endometrium which are necessary for successful implantation to occur.
- *Sex hormone-binding globulin* (SHBG) is the specific binding globulin for testosterone and oestradiol. It is produced by the liver and has a molecular weight of about 100 000. Variations in the level of SHBG affect the amount of free steroid available and thus the biological activity of circulating oestradiol and testosterone. SHBG levels are decreased by androgens, in obesity and in hypothyroidism and are increased by oestrogens, in pregnancy and in hyperthyroidism.
- *Corticosterone-binding globulin* is the carrier globulin for progesterone and cortisol.

Hypothalamic–pituitary–ovarian cycle (see Figure 3.1)

- *FSH* stimulates the development of many follicles most of which undergo atresia at different stages. One or more dominant follicles continues to grow each cycle and produces increasing amounts of oestrogen.

- The *increasing oestradiol level* exerts a positive feedback effect on the production of FSH and LH by the pituitary. The effect on the release of the gonadotrophins is initially negative but, by a time and concentration-dependent effect, becomes positive and results in the midcycle LH surge.
- The *LH surge* causes ovulation to occur (approximately 36 hours later) followed by the formation of the corpus luteum which continues to secrete oestradiol and which secretes increasing quantities of progesterone.
- If pregnancy does not occur the corpus luteum degenerates, oestradiol and progesterone levels fall and menstruation ensues.
- Ovarian activity can be monitored using ultrasound. The dominant follicle is usually more than 20 mm in diameter prior to ovulation.

Endometrial cycle

- Following *menstruation* the basal endometrium is thin (0.5 mm), with narrow straight glands lined by cuboidal epithelium, and the stroma is compact.
- With *increasing oestrogen levels* the endometrial stroma and blood vessels proliferate. The epithelial cells lining the glands become taller with basally situated nuclei and the glands become longer but remain straight. By midcycle the endometrium is 2–3 mm thick.
- As *progesterone levels increase* the glands become tortuous and convoluted. The nuclei in the glandular epithelium move towards the centre of the cell, as vacuoles form below the nucleus – subnuclear vacuolation. Secretions rich in glycogen, protein and fat accumulate in the glands reaching a maximum on about day 24.
- The stromal cells increase in size and the stroma becomes oedematous and the endometrium thickens to 5–6 mm.
- The arterioles become more and more coiled.
- As the *corpus luteum regresses* oestrogen and progesterone levels fall and the endometrium breaks down. The spiral arteries constrict and necrosis and bleeding occur; the superficial layers of the endometrium are shed with the menstrual flow.
- The duration of menstrual loss is usually less than a week.
- The average menstrual loss is 35 ml per period. More than 80 ml is considered excessive.
- Endometrial thickness can be measured using ultrasound.

Chapter 4

Puberty

The first signs of pubertal development in a girl normally occur between the ages of 9 and 13 years.

Tanner stages of puberty

Box 4.1 Tanner stages of puberty

Stage	*Age range* (years)	*Breast*	*Pubic hair*
1	Prepubertal	Elevation of nipple only	None
2	9–13	Breast bud begins to grow beneath nipple Areola enlarging	Sparse long pigmented hair on labia majora
3	10–14	Further enlargement of breast and areola in same contour	Sparse coarse hair over mons
4	11–15	Areola and nipple elevated above breast contour	Abundant adult type hair mainly limited to mons
5	12–17	Recession of areola to contour of breast	Hair of adult type and distribution

Peak height velocity is between stages 2 and 3. Menarche usually occurs during or after stage 4 and little further increase in height occurs after menarche

- Average age of menarche (first period) in developed countries is 12–14 years (normal range 10–16 years). Onset of menarche may be delayed by poor nutrition.
- Many changes occur in the years before the menarche.
- Normal course of events is commencement of breast development (thelarche) (Figure 4.1), development of pubic (Figure 4.2) and then axillary hair, maximum growth spurt and then menarche. Sequence can vary but menarche occurs only after some development in the above areas and only after there has been considerable breast development.
- Precise cause of onset of puberty is unknown. There is an increase in the adrenal production of dehydroepiandrosterone (DHEA) during childhood. The onset of puberty is associated with sleep-related increases in gonadotrophin levels. Ovarian follicular growth is stimulated and leads to increased oestrogen production causing breast development and eventually sufficient endometrial development to cause the first period to occur. Follicular cysts may be seen in the ovary on ultrasound scanning.

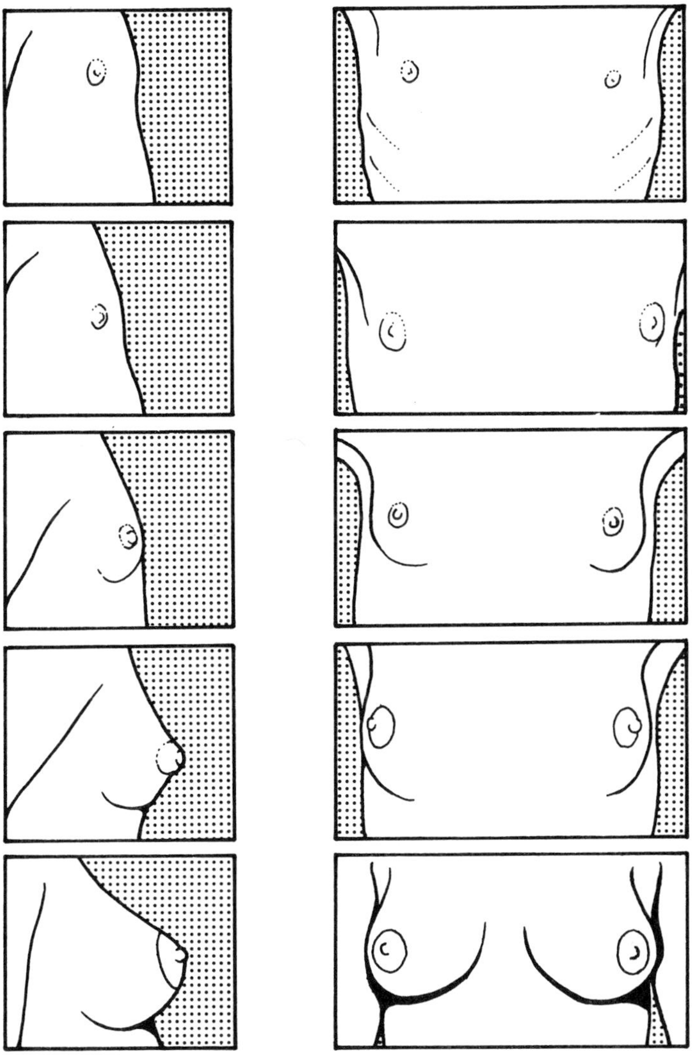

Figure 4.1 Tanner stages of puberty – breast development, stages 1–5.

- The first few periods are usually anovulatory, relatively painless and irregular. They then become regular and more painful as ovulatory cycles are established.

Problems associated with puberty and the menarche (Box 4.2)

Psychosocial problems

The transition from childhood through adolescence to adulthood is a time of anxiety for a girl and her mother. Anatomical, physiological and psychological changes occur that can be disturbing to the child unless handled sympathetically.

Box 4.2 Problems associated with puberty and the menarche

- Psychosocial problems
- Dysmenorrhoea (see Chapter 5)
- Heavy vaginal bleeding
- Infrequent periods that do not settle into a regular cycle – oligomenorrhoea (see Chapter 5)
- Delayed puberty
- Primary amenorrhoea (see Chapter 5)
- Precocious puberty

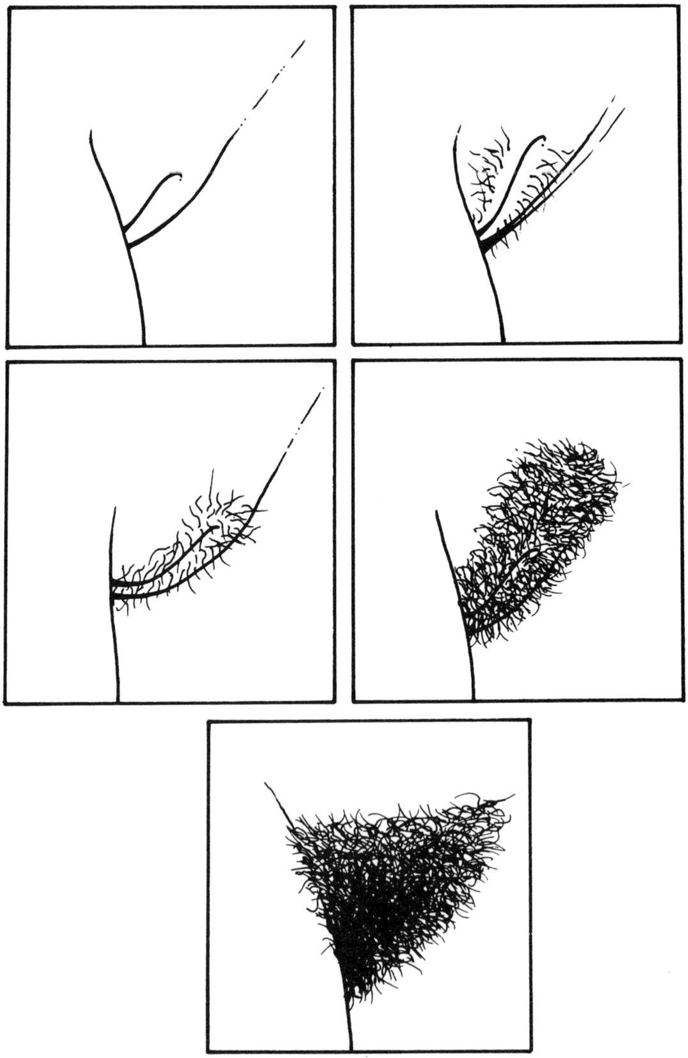

Figure 4.2 Tanner stages of puberty – pubic hair, stages 1–5.

- The girl should be made aware of the normal events of puberty and that these changes may occur at different ages in different girls. She may feel awkward and abnormal if the changes occur sooner in her peers than in herself and she should be reassured that this does not mean that she is abnormal.
- She also needs sympathetic help in the development of her independence and of new interests – particularly in her relationships with the family and with boys.

Dysmenorrhoea

For discussion of dysmenorrhoea see Chapter 5.

Heavy vaginal bleeding following the menarche

The first few periods are often anovulatory; they may be irregular and heavy because of unopposed oestrogen stimulation of the endometrium.

History

- A detailed history is important to establish whether the loss is in fact abnormal. The frequency, duration and protection required must be noted.

Management

- The reason for the heavy irregular bleeding should be explained to the girl and her mother and they should be reassured that the problem is usually self-limiting when ovulatory cycles commence.
- A menstrual chart should be kept.
- If the bleeding is unduly heavy a haemoglobin estimation should be made if necessary and the girl should be given iron and a progestogen. The progestogen can be given either alone in the form of dydrogesterone 10 mg twice daily from day 5 to 25 of the cycle or norethisterone 5–10 mg from day 10 to 25 of the cycle or in the form of a combined low dose oral contraceptive (particularly if the girl is sexually active). Treatment should be continued for 3–4 months and then stopped and a menstrual calendar kept.
- If the girl presents acutely with very heavy bleeding, this can usually be decreased and stopped by giving norethisterone up to 10 mg three times daily for 2–3 days, reducing gradually to 5 mg three times daily for a total of 20 days treatment and then recommencing in lower dosage in the next cycle.

Infrequent periods that do not settle into a regular cycle

- This may be indicative of an endocrine disorder such as the polycystic ovary syndrome (see Chapter 5).

Delayed puberty

Absence of pubertal development by 14 years of age or of menstruation by 16 years of age warrants investigation and appropriate management. Primary amenorrhoea is discussed in Chapter 5. For possible causes of delayed puberty see Box 4.3 and Figure 4.3.

Box 4.3 Possible causes of delayed puberty

- Constitutional (less than 3% by age of 14 years)
- Generalized disorders such as malnutrition, chronic illness, psychiatric problems (including anorexia nervosa or emotional deprivation) and weight or exercise-related hypogonadism
- Kallman's syndrome (associated with anosmia) and other hypothalamic disorders
- Hypothyroidism
- Several rare congenital conditions affecting one or more systems
- Ovarian dysgenesis usually associated with chromosome abnormality, e.g. XO (Turner's syndrome), one abnormal X-chromosome, mosaicism or XY gonadal dysgenesis. In these conditions LH and FSH levels will be elevated – hypergonadotrophic hypogonadism (see Chapter 5)

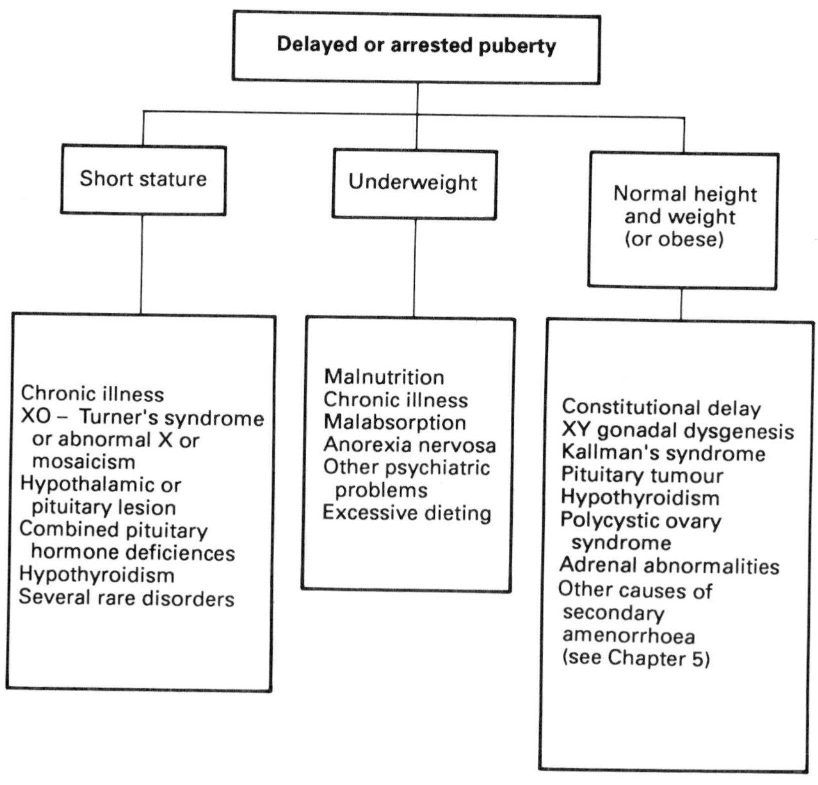

Figure 4.3 Delayed or arrested puberty.

Primary amenorrhoea

For a discussion of primary amenorrhoea see Chapter 5.

Precocious puberty

Precocious puberty implies pubertal changes beginning before the age of 8 years, or vaginal bleeding before the age of 10 years. For causes of precocious puberty see Box 4.4.

Box 4.4 Causes of precocious puberty

- Idiopathic and otherwise normal
- Abnormalities in CNS such as tumours, traumatic lesions or infections
- McCune–Albright syndrome (polyostotic fibrous dysplasia) – disseminated skeletal abnormalities and *café-au-lait* patches on skin
- Neurofibromatosis (von Recklinghausen's disease)
- Hypothyroidism
- Adrenal or ovarian tumours
- Drug ingestion, particularly oestrogens

Management

- This condition requires specialist evaluation and management by a paediatric endocrinologist.

Chapter 5

Amenorrhoea, menstrual problems and postmenopausal bleeding

It is very important that the terms used to describe abnormalities of the menstrual cycle are used appropriately. The following terms are in common use:

- Amenorrhoea

  Absence of menstruation.
  Primary amenorrhoea means that menstruation has never occurred.
  Secondary amenorrhoea means that menstruation has occurred in the past but not for at least 6 months.

- Oligomenorrhoea – periods occur less frequently than normal.
- Short cycles – the cycle length is less than 25 days.
- Short or inadequate luteal phase – luteal phase less than 10 days or progesterone level never reaches 30 nmol/l.
- Dysmenorrhoea – painful periods.
- Menorrhagia – heavy regular bleeding at approximately monthly intervals.
- Metropathia haemorrhagica – very heavy bleeding occurring after several weeks of amenorrhoea, associated with an anovulatory cycle. Due to unopposed oestrogen action from follicular development without ovulation.
- Intermenstrual bleeding – bleeding between periods.
- Postmenopausal bleeding

  Any bleeding from the genital tract more than 6 months after what had been considered to be the menopause.
  Any abnormal bleeding from the genital tract after what had been considered to be the menopause.

Other terms such as polymenorrhoea, epimenorrhoea and metromenorrhagia mean different things (or nothing) to different people and should not be used. If the patient's symptoms are not adequately covered by the accepted terms listed above they should be described in language that everyone can understand, e.g. continuous bleeding for 3 weeks, bleeding for 5 days every 3 weeks.

Box 5.1 gives an example of history taking.

Amenorrhoea

Amenorrhoea is the absence of periods and may be physiological or pathological.

Box 5.1 Gynaecological history taking

Questions	*Possible answers as written in the notes*
Nature and duration of present complaint	Increasingly heavy periods for 2 years
Age (in years) at menarche	K 14
Duration of bleeding (days)	$\frac{7}{28}$
Cycle length (number of days from first day of one period to first day of next period)	
Number of tampons and pads per period	No tampons, 40 pads
Pain with periods	Moderate discomfort for first 2 days
Bleeding between periods	No IMB (intermenstrual bleeding)
Bleeding after intercourse	No PCB (postcoital bleeding)
Discharge	No discharge
Contraception	Diaphragm
Past gynaecological history	Nil of note. Last smear 2 years ago
Past obstetric history	C_2 – aged 8 years FTND (full term normal delivery) – aged 5 years FTND
Past medical and surgical history	Nil of note

Physiological amenorrhoea

- Premenarchial.
- Pregnancy.
- Puerperal.
- Postmenopausal.

Pathological amenorrhoea

- Primary amenorrhoea – no periods have ever occurred. More than 95% of normal girls start menstruating by the age of 16 years.
- Secondary amenorrhoea – absence of menstruation for 6 months or more.

For menstruation to occur there must be normal hypothalamic, pituitary, ovarian and uterine function and a patent cervix and vagina. There may be an abnormality at any of these levels or amenorrhoea may be due to external influences.

Primary amenorrhoea

For the aetiology of primary amenorrhoea see Box 5.2.

Primary amenorrhoea at 14 years of age

If a girl presents at the age of 14 years with primary amenorrhoea, a full history should be taken and a general and vulval examination should be performed. Height and weight should be noted.

Box 5.2 Aetiology of primary amenorrhoea

Hypothalamus

- Kallman's syndrome (congenital failure of LHRH production associated with anosmia)(1)
- Anorexia nervosa (2)
- Hypothalamic amenorrhoea (associated with weight loss, emotional trauma, excessive exercise etc.)(2)
- Hypothalamic tumour or trauma (2)

Pituitary

- Tumour (2)

Gonads

- Streak gonads
  - XO Turner's syndrome (1, rarely 2)
  - XX or mosaic (1, rarely 2)
  - XY gonadal dysgenesis (1)
- Testicular feminization (1)
- Polycystic ovary syndrome (2)
- Hermaphroditism (1)

Uterus

- Absent (müllerian agenesis) – often associated with renal abnormality (1)
  – testicular feminization (1)

Vagina

- Absent (1)
- Cryptomenorrhoea due to imperforate hymen (1) (see Chapter 17)

External influences

- Weight loss due to generalized disease or anorexia nervosa (2)
- Drugs (2)
- Endocrine disorders – diabetes, adrenal and thyroid abnormalities (2)

(1) Cause of primary amenorrhoea only
(2) Also a cause of secondary amenorrhoea

Note: Other conditions that cause secondary amenorrhoea may also cause primary amenorrhoea

---

- Check that ponderal index [weight in kg/(height in m)^2] is normal.
- If there are no signs of puberty investigate and manage as for delayed puberty (see Chapter 4).
- If there are signs of puberty determine the stage and check that the vaginal orifice is patent by inspection.

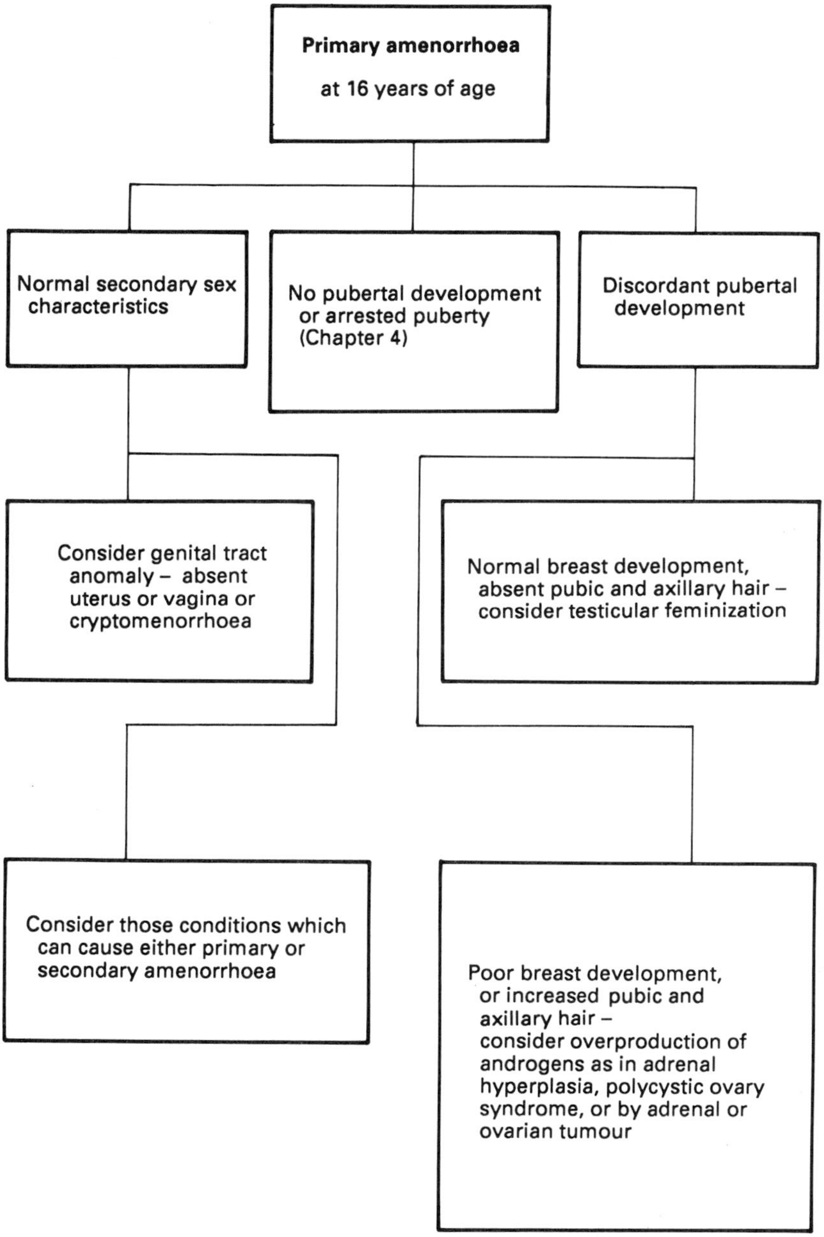

Figure 5.1 Primary amenorrhoea.

- Exclude obvious endocrine abnormalities and review in a few months to ensure that pubertal development is progressive.

Primary amenorrhoea at 16 years of age (Figure 5.1)

If a girl presents at the age of 16 years with primary amenorrhoea detailed investigation is appropriate because there is an increasing risk of malignancy if the gonads are not removed in a girl with a Y-chromosome.

History and examination

A full history should be taken and a general and vulval examination performed.

Investigations

These will depend on the findings in the history and examination but will include some of the following:

- *Chromosome analysis* from a peripheral blood sample.
- *FSH and LH* – to distinguish between hypergonadotrophic (gonadal dysgenesis), eugonadotrophic and hypogonadotrophic hypogonadism.
- *Prolactin* – to detect hyperprolactinaemia.
- *T_4 and TSH* – to diagnose thyroid disorders.
- *Lateral skull X-ray* – to detect abnormalities of the pituitary fossa and abnormal areas of calcification.
- *Other investigations* are arranged as appropriate, e.g. measurement of androgen levels if there is hirsutism.

Sex chromosome abnormalities

XO (Turner's syndrome), deleted arm(s) of X or mosaic (e.g XX/XO)

- Patient will usually be of short stature (less than 5 feet or 152 cm) and there will often be somatic abnormalities such as a web neck, shield-shaped chest and increased carrying angle and, sometimes, cardiovascular abnormalities.
- External and internal genitalia are normal.
- Where there is gonadal agenesis there is no pubertal development and LH and FSH are high (hypergonadotrophic hypogonadism), unless hormonal treatment has been given. In a few patients with Turner's syndrome or mosaicism there may be some functioning ovarian tissue.
- Chromosome analysis will enable a diagnosis to be made.

Management

- Full discussion with patient and parents about significance of the condition.
- Oestrogen replacement therapy is indicated in patients with streak gonads up until the age of 50 years or more to produce secondary sexual development, to prevent symptoms of oestrogen deficiency and to reduce likelihood of development of osteoporosis. Combined oestrogen and progestogen therapy is indicated after 1 or 2 years to protect the endometrium against unopposed oestrogen. (Ethinyl oestradiol 10 μg once a day for 21 out of 28 days for 6 months to a year, then 20 μg once a day for 21 out of 28 days for 6 months to a year and then cyclical combined oestrogen and progestogen therapy, e.g. ethinyl oestradiol 35 μg and norethisterone 500 μg for 21 out of every 28 days.)
- Review every 4 months to check progress and then when established satisfactorily on cyclical combined oestrogen and progestogen therapy review annually.

- Explain that pregnancies have been achieved in several women with non-functioning gonads by ovum donation with hormonal support of early pregnancy, using *in vitro* fertilization or related techniques, and that further improvements in these techniques are likely.
- As long as no Y-chromosome is present, gonadectomy is not indicated.

XY gonadal dysgenesis

- The presence of a Y-chromosome is associated with a markedly increased risk of gonadal malignancy and so bilateral gonadectomy should be performed.
- Subsequent management with hormone replacement therapy and possibilities for pregnancy are the same as in Turner's syndrome.

XY testicular feminization

- Familial.
- In this condition, müllerian duct development is suppressed by müllerian inhibiting factor produced by the testes which are usually intra-abdominal. The uterus and tubes are therefore absent and the vagina is short and blind.
- There is insensitivity to the testosterone produced by the testes but the tissues respond to oestrogen and so there is good breast development.
- Bilateral gonadectomy is indicated because of the risk of malignancy. Oestrogen replacement therapy should be started immediately because otherwise gonadectomy will precipitate acute menopausal symptoms.

Secondary amenorrhoea

Box 5.3 Aetiology of secondary amenorrhoea

Physiological

- Pregnancy
- Lactation
- Menopause

Hypothalamic

- Anorexia nervosa
- Hypothalamic amenorrhoea (associated with weight loss, stress, emotional trauma, excessive exercise etc.)
- Drugs (e.g. phenothiazines)
- Hypothalamic tumour or trauma, craniopharyngioma
- Pseudocyesis

Pituitary

- Tumour – usually prolactin secreting but may occur with other pituitary tumours
- Failure – Sheehan's syndrome (postpartum pituitary necrosis) or other forms of pituitary failure

Box 5.3 *continued*

Ovaries

- Polycystic ovary syndrome
- Ovarian failure (premature menopause)
- Resistant ovary syndrome
- Hormone-secreting ovarian tumours
- Oophorectomy

Uterus

- Pregnancy
- Asherman's syndrome (intrauterine adhesions)
- Hysterectomy

Cervix

- Obliteration of canal following cautery, cone biopsy or amputation of cervix at time of repair operation

External influences

- Weight loss due to generalized disease
- Drugs
- Endocrine disorders, e.g. diabetes, adrenal and thyroid abnormalities

Box 5.4 History from patient with secondary amenorrhoea

- Age at menarche?
- Pattern of cycles?
- Duration of amenorrhoea?
- Pregnancy symptoms?
- Weight loss?
- Severe illness?
- Drugs, including contraceptive pill?
- Emotional trauma?
- Exercise?
- Hirsutism?
- Galactorrhoea?
- Hot flushes?
- Polydipsia?
- Polyuria?
- Previous pregnancies?
- Operations?
- Physical trauma, e.g. head injury?
- Abnormality of visual fields?

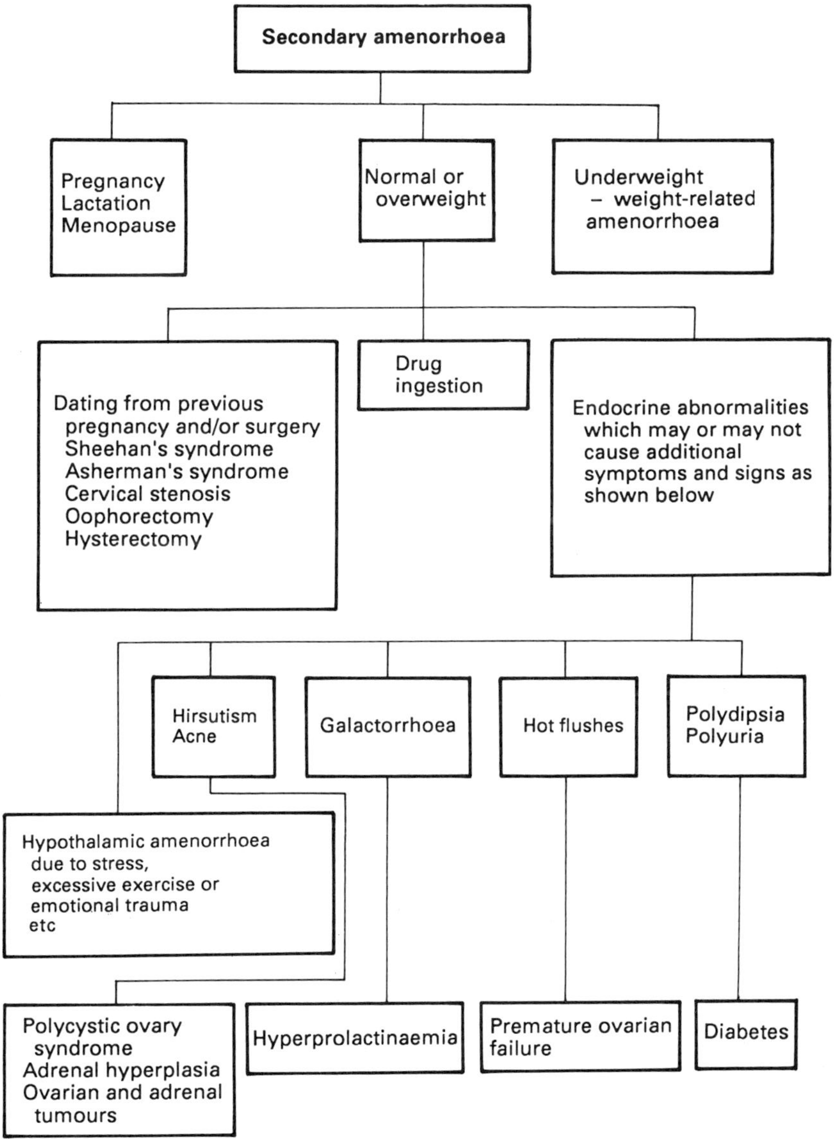

Figure 5.2 Secondary amenorrhoea.

Management of secondary amenorrhoea

If amenorrhoea is of short duration and no abnormality is found in the history or on examination of a young woman, no investigation is necessary as the problem is usually self-limiting. Arrange to review if amenorrhoea persists beyond 1 year. Earlier investigation is appropriate in an older woman (25–40 years) or if pregnancy is desired.

Investigations

Depending on history and examination some or none of the following investigations may be appropriate:

- *FSH and LH* – raised in ovarian failure and resistant ovary syndrome. LH:FSH ratio often increased in polycystic ovary syndrome.
- *Prolactin* – raised in hyperprolactinaemia, in hypothyroidism and with drugs that interfere with dopamine action, e.g. phenothiazines, reserpine.
- *T_4 and TSH* – if thyroid dysfunction suspected or hyperprolactinaemia detected.
- *Testosterone* – raised in polycystic ovary syndrome and with androgen secreting tumour
- *Sex hormone-binding globulin* – decreased in polycystic ovary syndrome, hypothyroidism and obesity.
- *Lateral skull X-ray* if pituitary tumour suspected.
- *Ultrasound* to confirm pregnancy or polycystic ovary syndrome, if necessary.

Treatment

Any significant non-gynaecological abnormality (such as low body weight or diabetes) will require treatment in its own right.

Hypothalamic amenorrhoea

If there is no significant abnormality in the history, examination and investigations (including normal LH, FSH and prolactin levels) and the patient wishes to become pregnant, ovulation induction with clomiphene citrate is indicated. Treatment is started with 50 mg once a day for 5 days and is repeated from day 3 of the period if the treatment is successful. If no follicular development occurs with 50 mg increase to 100 mg for 5 days. If follicular development (detected by an increase in oestradiol level after 10 days or by ultrasound) occurs but not ovulation HCG 5000 or 10 000 units should be given 5 days after the end of the course of clomiphene citrate. If no response to clomiphene citrate, consider treatment with gonadotrophins or LHRH infusion if adequate hormonal and ultrasound surveillance available.

Hyperprolactinaemia

- Repeat estimation under ideal conditions to confirm diagnosis. Note that prolactin levels are raised during stress, suckling, intercourse, sleep and general anaesthesia.
- Exclude drug intake and hypothyroidism and then investigate with visual field assessment, lateral skull X-ray and computerized tomography (CT) scan.
- For a microadenoma, bromocriptine is the treatment of choice. Start with 1.25 mg (half a tablet) after supper, as it can cause nausea and hypotension if taken without

food. Increase to 2.5 mg after supper and then 2.5 mg twice a day with food (average dose) if necessary.

- Prolactin level will fall to normal within a few hours of adequate dose of bromocriptine and will increase as soon as treatment discontinued. Menstruation should resume within 2 months.
- Repeat prolactin estimation in 2–3 months and review with result. If suppression inadequate, dose may need to be increased. Once stabilized arrange regular follow-up every 4–6 months.
- Advise patient to discontinue bromocriptine once pregnancy confirmed.

Premature ovarian failure

- If FSH and LH markedly raised (>20 units/litre), the most likely diagnosis is ovarian failure but can be due to resistant ovary syndrome in which the ovary is temporarily resistant to endogenous gonadotrophin stimulation.
- FSH and LH estimation should be repeated and cause for ovarian failure sought (e.g. previous radiotherapy).
- Hormone replacement therapy should be prescribed for women with premature ovarian failure.
- Successful pregnancies have been achieved with ovum donation and hormonal support of early pregnancy.
- Currently, no known treatment for resistant ovary syndrome but spontaneous resolution may occur.

Polycystic ovary syndrome

If hirsute, and testosterone and LH raised and FSH normal, polycystic ovary syndrome is likely (see Box 5.5 for details).

Oligomenorrhoea

'Oligomenorrhoea' is a term usually used to mean infrequent periods; it often dates from the menarche.

Aetiology

- Frequently associated with the polycystic ovary syndrome.
- Sometimes related to another endocrine disorder, such as hyperprolactinaemia, thyroid dysfunction, diabetes or adrenal hyperplasia.
- Several of the other factors which can cause secondary amenorrhoea may cause oligomenorrhoea (Box 5.3).
- Sometimes idiopathic.

Box 5.5 Polycystic ovary syndrome

- Common disorder, usually presents with oligomenorrhoea and hirsutism dating from the menarche
- Obesity is often but not always present

Diagnosis

This can usually be made from history and examination

Examination

- Usually hirsute
- Ovaries may be palpably enlarged to two to three times normal size on vaginal examination

Investigations (not all necessary)

- Testosterone raised (two to three times normal female level)
- Sex hormone-binding globulin (SHBG) lowered
- Free testosterone raised
- LH usually raised, FSH normal (ratio usually >2.5:1)
- Polycystic ovaries can be diagnosed on ultrasound with typical appearance of multiple small (<5 mm diameter) cysts round the periphery of the ovaries, i.e. necklace appearance

Treatment

- Subfertility – clomiphene citrate 50–100 mg a day for 5 days from day 3 of period. If this causes follicular development, detected by rise in oestradiol level or by ultrasound, but not ovulation then give HCG 5000 or 10 000 units 5 days after clomiphene citrate or when follicle mature on ultrasound examination. If no response to clomiphene citrate, gonadotrophin treatment can be considered but there is an increased risk of hyperstimulation and multiple pregnancy. LHRH infusion is not particularly effective. Suppression of LH with LHRH agonist followed by gonadotrophin treatment may be beneficial
- Hirsutism and/or contraception:
  (1) Oestrogenic contraceptive pills (such as Brevinor and Ovysmen – ethinyl oestradiol 35 μg and norethisterone 500 μg) suppress LH (which stimulates ovarian androgen production), and increase SHBG and therefore reduce free testosterone
  (2) Diane and Dianette contain the anti-androgen cyproterone acetate as well as ethinyl oestradiol and may be helpful in controlling hirsutism
- Anovulatory amenorrhoea – cyclical progestogen therapy to protect endometrium against unopposed oestrogen stimulation (e.g. norethisterone 5–10 mg or medroxyprogesterone acetate 5 mg from day 10 to 25 of cycle) should be considered

Management

- Consider possible endocrine disorder by careful history, examination and investigation.
- *History* – similar to that for secondary amenorrhoea (see Box 5.4).
- *Examination* – note particularly height and weight, presence or absence of hirsutism and galactorrhoea; examine the thyroid and perform a vaginal examination.

Investigation

- If hirsute, testosterone and sex hormone-binding globulin levels, LH and FSH.
- If galactorrhoea, prolactin level and, if hyperprolactinaemia or if suspicion of thyroid disorder, thyroid function tests.
- Check urine for glucose.
- Ovarian ultrasound may occasionally be indicated.

Treatment

- If a cause is found this will usually require specific treatment.
- If no cause found and the patient is infertile and wishes to become pregnant (and the weight is normal), clomiphene citrate 50 mg a day for 3 days from day 3 of the period is the initial treatment of choice, increasing to 50 mg and then 100 mg for 5 days if necessary, with the addition of HCG if indicated (see above).
- If pregnancy not desired cyclical progestogen therapy should be considered because of the long-term risk of endometrial carcinoma in women with persistently anovulatory cycles. Barrier contraception can be used or a combined contraceptive pill can be prescribed.

Short cycles

- Cycle length less than 25 days.
- May be anovulatory or due to short luteal phase.
- Important to distinguish between truly short cycles and intermenstrual bleeding.
- Condition may be self-limiting. Common in perimenopausal years.

Management

- If history unclear, menstrual chart may be helpful.
- If just short cycles (and not intermenstrual bleeding) and pregnancy not desired, a progestogen, e.g. norethisterone 5 mg once or twice daily can be given from day 10 to 25 of the cycle.
- If desiring pregnancy, a temperature chart should be kept – if cycles anovular look for a cause (see above); if short luteal phase, see below.

Short or inadequate luteal phase

- The normal luteal phase lasts 10–14 days and there should be a sustained rise in basal body temperature due to progesterone production by the corpus luteum.
- Plasma progesterone should be greater than 30 nmol/l between 8 and 6 days before a period, i.e. 6–8 days after ovulation.

- A short or inadequate luteal phase may be due to a general endocrine disorder or to hypothalamic–pituitary–ovarian dysfunction. If no cause is found and pregnancy is desired clomiphene citrate 50 mg once a day for 3 days from day 3 of period may improve follicular development and corpus luteum function. Ultrasound monitoring may be helpful.

Dysmenorrhoea

- Means pain with periods – may be primary or secondary.
- Is a very common problem – most women have dysmenorrhoea at some time in their lives.

Primary dysmenorrhoea

- Usually dates from soon after menarche with onset of ovulatory cycles.
- Is not associated with organic disease.
- Starts just before onset of period and usually lasts for less than 24 hours.
- Is colicky and is felt centrally in lower abdomen but may radiate to back and thighs.
- May be accompanied by other symptoms such as nausea, vomiting, diarrhoea and fainting.
- Some of the symptoms are due to prostaglandin release.
- Usually diminishes in severity with increasing age.

Treatment

- Important to identify any psychosocial factors which may aggravate the symptoms.
- Simple analgesics are sufficient treatment in many cases.
- Prostaglandin synthetase inhibitors such as mefenamic acid 250–500 mg three times daily from the start of the period, until the pain subsides, may be helpful.
- Suppression of ovulation with a combined contraceptive pill will almost always be beneficial.
- A progestogen alone (such as dydrogesterone 10 mg twice a day from day 5 to 25 of the cycle) may be helpful when contraception is not required or if oestrogens are contraindicated. This preparation is non-masculinizing and is thought not to have any deleterious effects on a developing embryo.

Secondary dysmenorrhoea

- Starts later in life than primary dysmenorrhoea.
- Is usually related to pelvic congestion or organic disease such as endometriosis, pelvic inflammatory disease, adenomyosis or fibroids or may be due to retrograde bleeding along the fallopian tubes into the peritoneal cavity.

- Backache and lower abdominal discomfort may start several days before the period and may continue throughout the period.
- A fibroid polyp is an uncommon but important cause of secondary dysmenorrhoea.

Diagnosis

- Important to enquire about other symptoms such as dyspareunia, infertility and menorrhagia and to obtain psychosocial history.
- Vaginal examination is essential and may reveal features of endometriosis, pelvic inflammatory disease, adenomyosis, fibroids or psychosexual dysfunction.
- Laparoscopy may be required to confirm or exclude demonstrable pathology.

Treatment

- A sympathetic, supportive approach is helpful.
- If an organic cause is found appropriate treatment should be given (see relevant chapter).
- If no organic cause is found, psychosexual evaluation with appropriate treatment is often beneficial.
- Some women will demand a hysterectomy but this will often be followed by further pelvic symptoms if preoperative psychosexual evaluation is inadequate.

Menorrhagia

This is the term used for heavy regular periods:

- Women vary enormously in their description and tolerance of vaginal bleeding. It is therefore very important, although often difficult, to try to find out whether the bleeding is in fact abnormally heavy. Some women intentionally exaggerate their symptoms and others minimize them to a surprising degree. In a doubtful case, it may be necessary to see the woman when the bleeding is said to be heavy.
- Average menstrual loss is 35 ml per period. Menorrhagia implies a blood loss greater than 80 ml per period.
- Heavy bleeding cannot be controlled with tampons alone, with only one sanitary pad at a time or without having to get up at night to change tampons and pads.
- Menorrhagia will often lead to iron deficiency anaemia and a haemoglobin estimation should be performed.

Aetiology (Figure 5.3)

Local causes

- Leiomyomas (fibroids).
- Adenomyosis.

- Congenital uterine anomaly (e.g. bicornuate uterus).
- Intrauterine contraceptive device.
- Endometrial polyp.
- Endometrial carcinoma.
- Pelvic inflammatory disease.

General causes

- Idiopathic (dysfunctional uterine bleeding).
- Hypothyroidism.
- Coagulation disorder (such as thrombocytopenic purpura or von Willebrand's disease) or occasionally anticoagulant therapy.

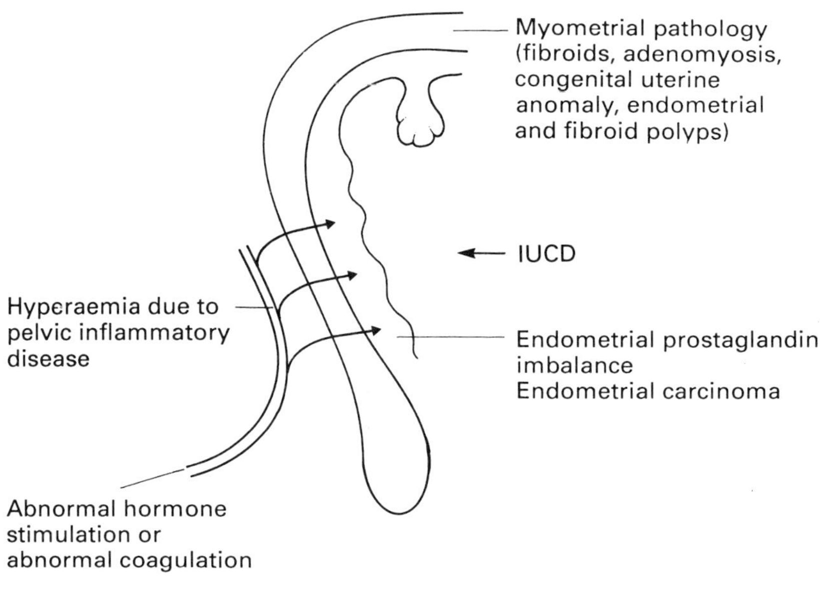

Figure 5.3 Some causes of menorrhagia.

Management

- General and gynaecological history.
- Try to assess severity of blood loss and enquire specifically for other symptoms such as intermenstrual bleeding and dysmenorrhoea.
- General and gynaecological examination.

Investigation

- Depends on findings in history and on examination and on severity of symptoms and age of patient.

- If there is intermenstrual bleeding as well as menorrhagia or if the bleeding is very heavy, or if the patient is more than 35 years of age, diagnostic curettage (Box 5.6) will usually be indicated, preceded by hysteroscopy if available, if no cause for the menorrhagia is identified.

Box 5.6 Diagnostic curettage

- Frequently performed procedure
- Main indications are menorrhagia, intermenstrual and postmenopausal bleeding
- Can be performed under general anaesthesia or with local anaesthetic, e.g. paracervical block
- Sterile precautions, clean and drape patient
- Catheterization seldom necessary
- Bimanual examination to assess size and position of uterus and to exclude cervical and adnexal abnormalities
- Speculum inserted and cervix and vagina inspected
- Cervix grasped with volsellum, length of uterine cavity measured with sound (normal length approximately 7 cm)
- Cervix (canal and internal os) dilated to 8–10 mm
- Polyp forceps introduced along full length of cavity in anteroposterior diameter, opened, closed and turned through 180° and withdrawn and then re-introduced in transverse diameter and opened, closed, turned through 180° and withdrawn
- Curettage performed – anterior wall, posterior wall, lateral walls and across fundus
- All tissue obtained sent for histological examination
- Monitor pulse and blood pressure on return to ward
- Patient may go home, accompanied, after 6 hours if all is well
- Warn her that she may have erratic bleeding for several days and that her next period may not be representative of future periods

Treatment

- If a cause is found then appropriate specific treatment is given.
- If no cause can be found empirical medical treatment can be tried – this can be either non-hormonal or hormonal.

Non-hormonal medical treatment

- Prostaglandin synthetase inhibitors, such as mefenamic acid 500 mg three times daily, from onset of bleeding.
- Antifibrinolytic agents may occasionally be of value but are not often used because of their side-effects.

Hormonal treatment

- Cyclical combined oral contraceptive pill with reasonable amount of progestogen such as Gynovlar (50 μg ethinyl oestradiol + 3 mg norethisterone), or Brevinor or

Ovysmen (35 μg ethinyl oestradiol + 500 μg norethisterone) with added extra norethisterone, e.g. 5 mg once daily from day 10 to 25 if necessary.

- If oestrogens contraindicated (e.g. in older women), progestogens can be given alone, e.g. norethisterone 5 mg twice or three times daily from day 5 or 10 to day 25 of cycle.
- Danazol can be given continuously 200 mg once daily, but essential to ensure conception does not occur. Side-effects are often unacceptable.

Surgical treatment

- Diagnostic curettage may also be therapeutic and will reassure the patient that her symptoms are not due to cancer if histology is benign (Box 5.7).

Box 5.7 Histology of curettings in menorrhagia

- Appropriate for day of cycle – treat as indicated above
- Cystic endometrial hyperplasia (due to anovulation) – treat with progestogen as above
- Atypical hyperplasia (a premalignant change) – treat by hysterectomy or, in a young woman, cyclical progestogen therapy for 4–6 months followed by repeat curettage can be tried

- Hysterectomy may be appropriate but the decision should not be taken hastily, particularly in the absence of demonstrable pathology and/or clear-cut menorrhagia, because there may be underlying social or psychosexual problems which will not be resolved by hysterectomy (Box 5.8).

Metropathia haemorrhagica

- Very heavy bleeding after several weeks of amenorrhoea, associated with anovulatory cycles.
- Usually occurs at extremes of reproductive life – at time of the menarche or, most commonly, perimenopausally.
- Follicular development occurs and continues as ovulation fails to take place. This results in high circulating unopposed oestrogen levels which continue to stimulate endometrial development causing cystic glandular hyperplasia.
- Eventually, after several weeks the endometrium breaks down and prolonged heavy bleeding occurs.

Diagnosis

- History.
- Diagnostic curettage – bulky curettings show cystic glandular hyperplasia on histological examination.

Box 5.8 Abdominal hysterectomy

Terms used

- Total hysterectomy to gynaecologist means removal of whole of uterus (corpus and cervix), but to patient may mean removal of uterus and ovaries
- Subtotal hysterectomy means removal of corpus but not cervix; seldom performed except where there would be considerable technical difficulty in removing the cervix (as in severe endometriosis) or in a postpartum hysterectomy

Counselling

- Decision to perform hysterectomy for a benign condition should only be made after full discussion of advantages and disadvantages and of alternative modes of treatment, particularly in a woman under 40 years of age
- Important to make clear what a hysterectomy will and will not achieve. Thus if ovaries are conserved premenstrual symptoms, if any, will continue

Preoperative investigations– as for any major operation

Postoperative care

- As for any major operation
- Watch for urinary retention
- Discuss histological findings appropriately

Advice on discharge from hospital

- Convalescence with minimal activity for 2 weeks followed by gradual resumption of household activities over next 4 weeks
- No intercourse for 6 weeks
- Check-up at 6 weeks includes history, examination of wound and speculum examination; there may be granulation tissue at the vault which can be cauterized with silver nitrate
- Return to full activities by 2–3 months after operation

Treatment

- Cyclical progestogen therapy, e.g. norethisterone 5–10 mg once daily from day 10 to 25 of the cycle.

Intermenstrual bleeding

It is necessary to find out amount of bleeding and when it occurs. It is an important symptom with several possible serious underlying causes and it must always be adequately investigated (Box 5.9).

History

This may be helpful in the differential diagnosis. Vaginal examination is essential and further investigation is often required:

- *Postcoital bleeding* is bleeding that occurs after intercourse. Usually due to local lesion such as cervical ectropion, polyp or carcinoma, or atrophic vaginitis.
- *Midcycle bleeding* may occur around time of ovulation due to slight fall in oestrogen levels that precedes ovulation.
- *Premenstrual spotting* may be due to inadequate hormone production by the corpus luteum.
- *Breakthrough bleeding* may occur in a woman taking the Pill if the composition of the Pill is inappropriate for that woman or Pill taking is erratic.

Box 5.9 Causes of intermenstrual bleeding

Cervical lesions

- Ectropion
- Polyp
- Carcinoma

Uterine lesions

- Endometrial polyp
- Related to intrauterine contraceptive device
- Endometrial carcinoma
- Fibroid polyp

Fallopian tube

- Carcinoma of fallopian tube (rare)
- Hormonal problems
- Ovulation bleeding
- Premenstrual spotting
- Breakthrough bleeding in woman taking the pill

Important to exclude bleeding arising outside the genital tract, e.g. bleeding from urinary and alimentary tracts

Diagnosis

- Speculum examination of the vagina and cervix is mandatory.
- A cervical smear should usually be taken.
- Diagnostic curettage will often be indicated.

Treatment

- The treatment is that of the cause.

Postmenopausal bleeding (PMB)

- Any bleeding from the genital tract more than 6 months after what had been considered to be the menopause.

- Any abnormal bleeding from the genital tract after what had been considered to be the menopause.
- Important to be sure that the bleeding is from the genital and not from the urinary or alimentary tracts. Good history essential – if any doubt remains appropriate investigation of the urinary or alimentary tracts may be indicated.

Causes of postmenopausal bleeding from the genital tract

Vulva

Postmenopausal bleeding is very rarely vulval in origin although a urethral caruncle may present with bleeding; vulvitis and carcinoma of the vulva rarely present with bleeding.

Vagina

- Atrophic vaginitis due to decreased circulating oestrogen levels is common, but must not be definitively blamed for PMB until other causes have been excluded.
- Traumatic bleeding can occur due, for example, to attempted intercourse following abstinence. A crescentic tear in the posterior fornix may result.
- Vaginal ulceration can occur with ring pessary.
- Vaginal carcinoma is rare.

Cervix

- Cervical polyp.
- Squamous carcinoma of the cervix.
- Adenocarcinoma of the cervix (much less common).

Uterus

- Endometrial polyp.
- Endometrial carcinoma.
- Bleeding due to increased oestrogen levels either following oestrogen administration (hormone replacement therapy) or due to ovarian oestrogen-secreting tumour.

Fallopian tubes

- Carcinoma of the fallopian tube is rare but does occur and may cause a blood-stained vaginal discharge.

Ovaries

- Oestrogen-secreting ovarian tumour, such as thecoma or granulosa cell tumour.

Management

- Full history and general examination.
- Vaginal examination.
- Diagnostic curettage is usually indicated.

Treatment

- Is that of the cause.
- If other abnormalities have been excluded, atrophic vaginitis can be treated with intravaginal dienoestrol cream.

Heavy vaginal bleeding

The causes for heavy vaginal bleeding are given in Box 5.10.

Box 5.10 Causes of very heavy vaginal bleeding (haemorrhage) which may lead to patient being brought to hospital as an emergency

Gynaecological

- Incomplete abortion
- Menorrhagia
- Metropathia haemorrhagica
- Fibroid polyp
- Cervical carcinoma
- Secondary haemorrhage following hysterectomy, repair or cone biopsy
- Trauma – vulval and vaginal lacerations
- Trophoblastic tumour
- Cervical pregnancy

Obstetric

- Placenta praevia
- Placental abruption
- Primary or secondary postpartum haemorrhage

Chapter 6
Premenstrual syndrome

- Many women in the reproductive age group experience physical and/or psychological symptoms in the premenstrual phase of the cycle but only a small percentage seek medical help for this problem.
- The symptoms commence after ovulation and subside with the onset of bleeding.
- The symptoms are related to ovarian rather than to uterine function and will therefore continue after hysterectomy if the ovaries are conserved.
- There is often a background of stress, and unhurried sympathetic questioning is essential.
- Many symptoms are complained of, some of the most common are listed in Box 6.1.

Box 6.1 Common premenstrual (postovulatory symptoms)

Physical

- Bloatedness
- Weight gain
- Breast discomfort
- Headaches
- Backache
- Autonomic symptoms
- Skin disorders

Psychological

- Tension
- Irritability
- Aggression
- Moodiness
- Tearfulness
- Depression
- Lethargy
- Poor concentration
- Lack of confidence
- Poor coordination
- Restlessness
- Insomnia

Aetiology

- The aetiology is still unclear.
- Many hypotheses have been proposed relating to abnormalities in brain catecholamine levels, β-endorphin, α-melanocyte-stimulating hormone, prolactin, vasopressin and antidiuretic hormone secretion, oestrogen, progesterone, aldosterone and cortisol production, abnormalities in the renin angiotensin system, vitamin deficiencies etc.
- There is often a personal or family history of psychological problems.
- Placebo treatment is effective in approximately 50% of cases.

- A symptom chart kept for 3 or 4 months before treatment is helpful in demonstrating whether the symptoms are truly premenstrual or whether they occur throughout the cycle.
- Those that occur throughout the cycle or in a pattern unrelated to the cycle are not due to the premenstrual syndrome and a psychological/psychiatric cause for the symptoms should be sought.
- Those that occur only during the premenstrual fortnight are often exacerbated by psychological and stress factors.

Management (Figure 6.1)

- Essential to listen unhurriedly and sympathetically to the patient and to determine which symptoms are the most troublesome and whether there are any obvious precipitating causes.
- Obtain a general and social as well as a gynaecological and psychosexual history.
- Perform a general and vaginal examination and reassure the patient that she is normal if no abnormalities are found. Important that she knows that premenstrual symptoms are common and not indicative of serious underlying disease.
- If social or psychosexual problems are identified provide appropriate counselling.
- Ask the patient to keep a daily symptom and life event chart for 3–4 months to determine the nature and pattern of persistent symptoms and which, if any, occur only in the premenstrual fortnight.

Treatment

- *A placebo response* has been shown in approximately 50% of patients in double-blind trials with most medications that have been evaluated and a caring and sympathetic approach is certainly of great benefit and is often the most effective form of treatment.
- *Suppression of ovulation* – if the symptoms are truly due to the hormonal changes of the second half of the menstrual cycle they should be obliterated by suppression of ovulation. This can be achieved using a combined (oestrogen and progestogen) contraceptive pill taken cyclically. Continuous treatment with danazol or LHRH agonists has also been used but should be reserved for the severest cases as these drugs have profound side-effects.
- Other hormonal manipulations that have been found to be effective in some cases include progesterone suppositories (200–400 mg twice a day) or norethisterone 5–10 mg once a day in the second half of the cycle, dydrogesterone 20–40 mg once daily from day 5 or 12 to day 25 of the cycle, and an oestradiol implant coupled with an orally administered progestogen in the second half of the cycle.
- *Pyridoxine* (vitamin B_6) is an essential co-factor in the production of serotonin and of dopamine. Pyridoxine treatment is said to be particularly helpful when psychological or breast symptoms predominate but it should not be prescribed in high dosage over a prolonged period of time.

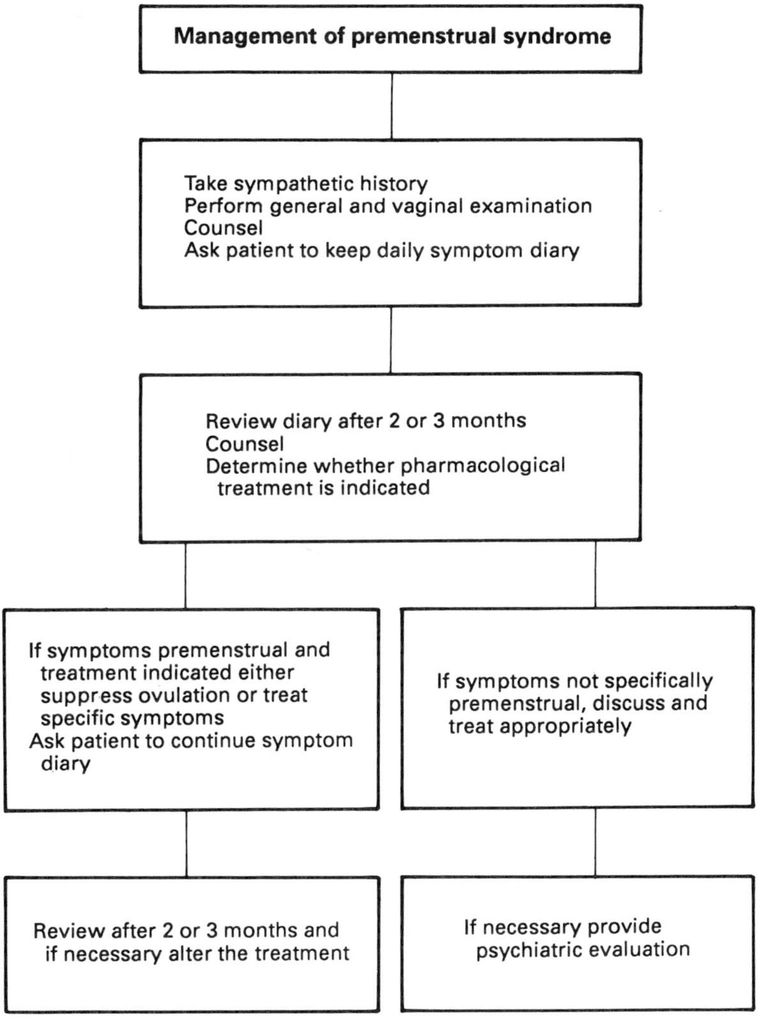

Figure 6.1 Management of premenstrual syndrome.

- Pyridoxine treatment can be combined with treatment with a progestogen in otherwise resistant cases.
- *Bromocriptine* (up to 2.5 mg twice daily) may be helpful when breast symptoms predominate.
- *A diuretic* taken for a few days each cycle may alleviate symptoms due to fluid retention.
- *Mefenamic acid* has been found to help some women particularly when headaches predominate.

The most important factor in helping the patient is to explore with her any possible causative factors and to provide sympathetic support and advice.

Chapter 7

Vaginal discharge and sexually transmitted diseases

Vaginal discharge

- Common complaint and may be physiological or due to local vaginal or cervical condition or occasionally to a problem higher in the genital tract.
- Patient often concerned that the discharge is due to venereal disease or to cancer.
- Likely diagnosis will depend on age of patient.

Local vaginal infections

- Vagina normally protected by apposition of its anterior and posterior walls, by well developed stratified epithelium and by low pH (3.5–4.5) due to production of lactic acid from glycogen by Döderlein's bacilli (lactobacilli). Poorly protected in children, puerperal and postmenopausal women.
- Vaginal infections are frequently sexually transmitted and a patient will often have more than one sexually transmitted disease at a time.

For the points to be noted in taking history and in examination of patients, see Box 7.2.

Candida albicans (monilia, thrush)

- Very common fungal infection.
- Grows well at pH 5–6.5, i.e. when vagina is less acid than normal.
- Increased incidence in reproductive age group, in pregnancy, in those taking antibiotics or on immunosuppressive therapy and in diabetics.

Clinical features

- May be asymptomatic.
- If causes discharge this is thick and white.
- Can cause severe itching, soreness and dyspareunia.
- On examination there may be white curds in the vagina with underlying redness and inflammation.
- Can affect vulva, intergluteal folds and inner aspects of thighs.

Box 7.1 Common causes of vaginal discharge in different age groups

Neonatal

- Clear or blood-stained discharge may occur for a few days after delivery due to fall in previously high oestrogen levels

Prepubertal

- Poor hygiene
- Chemical vulvovaginitis
- Vaginal infection
- Sexual interference
- Foreign body
- Worms

Puberty to menopause

- Normal physiological discharge, amount varies from woman to woman; some women find it hard to accept any discharge as normal
- Ovulatory mucus
- Local vaginal infection with *Candida albicans, Trichomonas vaginalis,* bacterial vaginosis or *Neisseria gonorrhoeae*
- Chemical vaginitis
- Foreign body
- Cervical lesions such as ectropion, polyp, carcinoma (discharge usually blood stained)
- Pelvic inflammatory disease due to, for example, *Chlamydia trachomatis, Neisseria gonorrhoeae, Mycoplasma hominis* – other symptoms usually present

Postmenopausal

- Atrophic vaginitis (discharge usually blood stained)
- Local vaginal infections as above
- Cervical lesions such as polyps or carcinoma (discharge usually blood stained)
- Endometrial polyps including fibroid polyps (discharge usually blood stained)
- Endometrial carcinoma (discharge usually blood stained)
- Carcinoma of fallopian tube – very rare
- Consider also urinary leak due to stress or urge incontinence, prolapse, and also rectal problems and fistulae

Diagnosis

- Microscopy may reveal mycelia and budding vegetative cells.
- Easily cultured in laboratory from swab placed in transport medium.
- May be identified in a cervical smear.

Box 7.2 Important points in history and examination of patient complaining of vaginal discharge

History

- Duration of discharge
- Amount
- Colour
- Consistency
- Odour
- Ever blood stained
- Associated symptoms such as itching and soreness
- Relationship to menstrual cycle
- Previous history of similar problem
- Previous history of sexually transmitted disease
- Any possible precipitating causes such as new sexual partner(s)

Examination

- *General examination* – exclude rash and examine mouth, if indicated
- *Abdominal examination* – any tenderness or masses
- *Vaginal examination* – inspect vulva, vagina, cervix and take urethral, vulval, high vaginal and cervical swabs, and cervical smear as appropriate, and then perform bimanual examination
- Place sample of discharge on a slide and add physiological saline and a coverslip and examine immediately under the microscope
- Send specimens to laboratory for microscopy and culture
- Syphilis serology if indicated
- Arrange for partner to be examined if indicated
- Colposcopy may be required
- If no cause found for symptoms re-evaluate psychosexual/social situation

Treatment

- Pessaries must be used and not just vulval creams as infection will persist in the vagina if vaginal treatment is not given.
- Clotrimazole (500 mg once at night or 200 mg for 3 nights or 100 mg for 6 nights) or nystatin pessaries (100 000 units for 14 nights). Disadvantage of nystatin is prolonged course required.
- Loose cotton rather than tight nylon underwear.
- Treat partner with cream if symptomatic or if infection recurs.
- If infection persists treat both partners with oral nystatin for one week to eradicate possible reservoir of infection in the bowel.
- Local gentian violet paint can be very effective but may cause a reaction.

Trichomonas vaginalis

- Very common protozoal infection.
- Usually but not always acquired by sexual contact.
- Important to treat both partners.

Clinical features

- May be asymptomatic.
- If produces discharge this is thin, frothy and greenish with unpleasant smell.
- Can cause intense itching, soreness and dyspareunia.
- On examination there is a frothy green discharge in the vagina which is reddend and rough.

Diagnosis

- Immediate microscopy of sample of discharge placed in drop of saline on a slide and covered with coverslip reveals pear-shaped motile flagellated protozoa.
- Can be cultured in laboratory from charcoal swab placed in transport medium.
- May be identified in a cervical smear.

Treatment

- Oral metronidazole (Flagyl) 200 mg three times daily for 7 days, 800 mg twice daily for 1 day or 2 g as a single dose.
- Sexual partner(s) should also be treated.
- Alcohol should not be taken during treatment as may cause flushing and severe headache.

Bacterial vaginosis

- Common condition associated with polymicrobial infection with the Gram-variable coccobacillus *Gardnerella vaginalis* (a facultative anaerobe), *Bacteroides* species (not *Bacteroides fragilis*) and other organisms.

Clinical features

- Often asymptomatic.
- If causes discharge this is profuse, adherent and grey in colour like thin flour paste.
- Strong fishy odour.
- Vaginal walls not inflamed.

Diagnosis

- Wet preparation shows abundance of 'clue' cells (squamous epithelial cells covered with masses of microorganisms).
- Vaginal pH $\geqslant$ 4.5.
- Fish odour increased by addition of potassium hydroxide to a drop of discharge in saline on a slide.

Treatment

- Metronidazole (Flagyl) 200 mg three times daily for 7 days for patient and partner.

Gonorrhoea

- Caused by Gram-negative diplococcus *Neisseria gonorrhoeae.*
- Common condition.
- Nearly always acquired by sexual contact – highly contagious.
- Infection occurs initially in the cervix and/or urethra and sometimes Bartholin's glands. Can also affect oropharynx and rectum.
- Contraceptive pill thickens cervical mucus and may prevent upward spread.

Clinical features

- Usually symptomatic in men but frequently asymptomatic in women and may persist for a long time.
- Incubation period usually 2–7 days but may be up to 2 months.
- If symptoms occur these are usually vaginal or urethral discharge and dysuria.
- Acute ascending infection may occur causing salpingitis, peritonitis and sometimes septicaemia, with skin lesions, arthritis and rarely endocarditis and perihepatitis (Fitz–Hugh–Curtis syndrome – see Box 7.3).

Diagnosis

- By microscopy and culture of cervical, urethral and rectal specimens; best plated out immediately or, if not possible, then send charcoal swabs in transport medium to laboratory.
- Blood culture if systemic infection suspected.
- Always perform serological (TPHA – *Treponema pallidum* haemagglutination) test for syphilis in patient with gonorrhoea.
- Exclude other sexually transmitted disease (approximately 50% of women with gonorrhoea also have *Chlamydia trachomatis* infection).

Treatment

- Oral ampicillin 3 g with probenecid 1 g.

- If organism resistant to penicillin, give cephalosporin with probenecid.
- If allergic to penicillin, give spectinomycin 2 g i.m.
- Repeat swabs one week later – no intercourse until swabs clear.
- Contacts must be traced and examined.

Long-term sequelae

If salpingitis occurs tubal damage is common and patient has increased risk of chronic pelvic inflammatory disease, ectopic pregnancy and infertility.

Box 7.3 Fitz–Hugh–Curtis syndrome

- Perihepatitis which occurs in about 10% of cases of pelvic inflammatory disease due to gonococcal or chlamydial infection
- Anorexia, nausea, vomiting
- Pain in right hypochondrium and shoulder tip pain from diaphragmatic irritation
- Positive Murphy's sign – tenderness in right hypochondrium
- Signs of peritonitis and pelvic infection
- Normal liver function tests

Chlamydia trachomatis

- Gram-negative obligate intracellular bacterium.
- Common infection.

Clinical features

- Often asymptomatic.
- May cause vaginal discharge.
- Is a common cause of pelvic inflammatory disease.
- Fitz–Hugh–Curtis syndrome may occur (Box 7.3).
- Important to ensure eradication before or during pregnancy because of risk of eye infection in neonates.

Diagnosis

- Can be made by culture from a swab placed in chlamydia transport medium (Figure 7.1) which has to be kept at 4°C and has a shelf life of 1–2 weeks.
- Immunofluorescent and enzyme immunoassay identification techniques are used in many centres. These may not be reliable for specimens from the pouch of Douglas and rectum.
- Serology generally unhelpful.

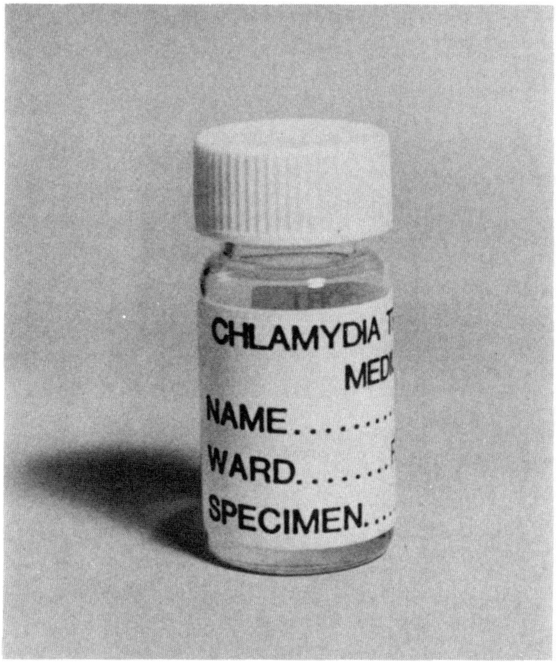

Figure 7.1 Chlamydia transport medium bottle.

- Exclude other sexually transmitted infections.

Treatment

- Tetracycline 500 mg 6-hourly for 1 week (not in pregnancy) or erythromycin stearate 500 mg 12-hourly for 2 weeks (in pregnancy).
- Repeat swabs 1 week later – no intercourse until swabs clear.
- Contacts must be traced and examined.

Long-term sequelae

This is a common cause of acute pelvic inflammatory disease which frequently leads to chronic pelvic inflammatory disease, risk of ectopic pregnancy and infertility.

Mycoplasma hominis

- Small Gram-negative rod, lacks bacterial cell wall.
- Common vaginal commensal in sexually active women.

Clinical features

- Often asymptomatic.

- Can cause pelvic inflammatory disease, postpartum genital tract infection and occasionally pyelonephritis.

Diagnosis

- Can be cultured from cervical swab (and occasionally from blood culture in postpartum infection).
- Interpret result with caution as may reflect normal flora.

Treatment

- Tetracycline or, if resistant, clindamycin.
- Not sensitive to erythromycin.

Chemical vaginitis

Vulvovaginal discomfort and sometimes discharge may be due to local reaction to chemicals in soap and washing powders, bath salts, douches or deodorants or to spermicides or condoms.

Foreign body

- Commonest foreign body in reproductive age group is a forgotten tampon, in older women a neglected ring pessary.
- Should be suspected in child with a persistent vaginal discharge.

Atrophic vaginitis

Vaginal discharge and discomfort in a postmenopausal woman is commonly due to atrophic vaginitis (see Chapter 17) and should be treated with oestrogen.

Cervical lesions causing vaginal discharge

Vaginal discharge may be due to a cervical ectropion or polyp (see Chapter 17) or to cervical carcinoma (see Chapter 20). In these conditions the discharge is frequently blood stained.

Vaginal discharge due to uterine and tubal pathology

- Endometrial polyps and carcinoma may present with a discharge but usually present with bleeding (see Chapters 17 and 20).
- Pelvic inflammatory disease may present with discharge but there are usually other symptoms as well as discussed later in this chapter.
- Carcinoma of the fallopian tube is very rare but it may present with a watery, often blood-stained, discharge (see Chapter 20).

Sexually transmitted diseases

- There are many sexually transmitted diseases and often more than one is present.
- Incidence of different infections varies in different parts of the world.
- May cause local or no symptoms or severe systemic disease.
- Commonly cause marital disharmony.
- Often best to refer patient with suspected sexually transmitted disease to department of genitourinary medicine for most efficient diagnosis, treatment and follow-up and because of their facilities for contact tracing.

Box 7.4 Sexually transmitted infections

- Trichomoniasis (see above)
- Gonorrhoea (see above)
- Chlamydial infection (see above)
- *Mycoplasma hominis* infection (see above)
- Genital herpes
- Human papilloma virus infection and genital warts
- Syphilis
- AIDS
- Chancroid
- Lymphogranuloma venereum
- Granuloma inguinale
- Other conditions such as candidiasis (see above), bacterial vaginosis (see above), pediculosis pubis and scabies are also frequently transmitted during sexual contact

Genital herpes

- Caused by herpes simplex viruses (types II and I).
- Highly contagious.

Clinical features

- May be asymptomatic.
- Symptoms usually appear within 7 days of contact.
- Usually causes very painful vesicular eruption on vulva which breaks down to form small ulcers that heal in about 2 weeks.
- Inguinal lymph nodes often enlarge.
- Recurrent attacks occur at irregular intervals.

Diagnosis

- May see multinucleated cells with dense chromatin and inclusion bodies in smear.
- Confirmed by culture of specimen (vesicular fluid or scrapings from ulcers) placed in viral transport medium and frozen at −70°C if not immediately cultured.

Treatment

- Analgesia and symptomatic treatment.
- Local treatment with idoxuridine or acyclovir.
- Acyclovir 200 mg orally 5 times a day for 7 days.

Human papilloma virus and genital warts (condylomata acuminata)

- Condylomata acuminata are caused by human papilloma virus (HPV).
- Some types of HPV (especially 16) have been implicated in the aetiology of cervical intraepithelial neoplasia and carcinoma.

Clinical features of genital warts

- Small warts which gradually increase in number on vulva, in vagina, on cervix and perianally.
- May form large soft friable lesions, especially during pregnancy or immunosuppressive treatment.

Diagnosis

- Macroscopic appearance.
- A cervical smear should be taken and the cervix should ideally be examined colposcopically.
- DNA hybridization test is under development.

Treatment

- If small and very few in number *and patient not pregnant* can be very carefully painted with podophyllin paint – painting must be very accurate and patient must be told to thoroughly wash the podophyllin off after 6 hours.
- May need diathermy under general anaesthetic or laser treatment.
- Treat partner.

Syphilis

- Caused by *Treponema pallidum* – a spirochaete.
- Nearly always acquired by sexual contact.

- Serious long-term sequelae and serious consequences for the baby if infected *in utero.*

Clinical features

- *Primary syphilis* – 9–90 days after contact a small papule appears and breaks down to form a solitary, shallow, punched out, painless ulcer (chancre) usually on cervix or labium, occasionally in mouth or on arms. Local lymph nodes enlarge and are rubbery, discrete and mobile and do not suppurate.
- *Secondary syphilis* – within a few weeks a symmetrical, copper-coloured, maculopapular rash, may appear on the trunk, limbs and occasionally the face; there may be generalized lymphadenitis, pyrexia, buccal ulceration, alopecia and iritis, and condylomata lata may appear on the vulva – these are flat topped, moist and necrotic. There may, however, be no manifestations of secondary syphilis.
- *Tertiary syphilis* – widespread manifestations occur due to involvement of the cardiovascular and central nervous systems and to the formation of gummata in any part of the body.

Diagnosis

- Dark ground examination of serum from primary chancre or condylomata lata will reveal white motile corkscrew-shaped spirochaetes.
- Serological conversion may take 3–4 weeks. False positives can occur.

Treatment

- Procaine penicillin 0.6 mega-units or 0.6 g daily for 10 days or tetracycline 2 g a day for 2 weeks.

Acquired immune deficiency syndrome (AIDS)

- Caused by human immunodeficiency virus (HIV).
- HIV can be transmitted from mother to fetus.

Clinical features

- Glandular fever like illness 4–6 weeks after infection in minority of cases.
- Latent phase of 2–5 years or more.
- Many modes of presentation due to opportunist infection (such as *Pneumocystis carinii* pneumonia etc.) or tumours (such as Kaposi's sarcoma) or to direct infection of cells (particularly in central nervous system) with HIV.

Diagnosis

- Can be confirmed by blood test, but seroconversion can take several months.

Treatment

- Supportive measures, because no specific treatment is available at the present time.

Chancroid (soft sore)

- Caused by *Haemophilus ducreyi* – a small Gram-negative rod.
- Mainly occurs in the Orient, West Indies and North Africa.

Clinical features

- Multiple small papules appear on vulva a few days after contact and quickly break down to form shallow, soft, irregular, painful ulcers containing purulent exudate and oedematous tissue.
- Inguinal nodes enlarged and tender and frequently suppurate (bubo).
- Malaise and pyrexia may occur but no other systemic effects.

Diagnosis

- Confirmed by culture of *Haemophilus ducreyi* from vulval discharge, swabs from ulcers or pus obtained by aspiration of inguinal node.

Treatment

- Co-trimoxazole or erythromycin.

Lymphogranuloma venereum

- Caused by different serotypes of *Chlamydia trachomatis* from those most commonly found in Europe.
- Mainly occurs in the Orient, Africa and South America.

Clinical features

- Papules appear 1–2 weeks after contact and break down in a few days to produce painless ulcers.
- With vulval lesion inguinal nodes are involved.
- With vaginal lesions pararectal lymph nodes discharge and break down forming sinuses.
- Scarring common causing rectal strictures.
- Damage to lymphatics causes lymphoedema.
- Malignant change occasionally occurs.

Diagnosis

- By culture from swabs placed in chlamydia transport medium (see above and Figure 7.1).

- By complement fixation test.

Treatment

- Bubos should be aspirated and not allowed to suppurate.
- Tetracycline or rifampicin and erythromycin.

Granuloma inguinale

- Caused by *Calymmatobacterium granulomatis* (Donovan's bacillus).
- Mainly occurs in the Tropics or subtropical zones.

Clinical features

- Painless papules appear days or months after contact and break down to form red granulomatous ulcers on vulva and in the groin.
- Inguinal lymph nodes may enlarge.
- Healing is by dense fibrosis with scarring.

Diagnosis

- Donovan bodies are seen in the cytoplasm of mononuclear cells, with Giemsa staining, in the exudate from the lesions.

Treatment

- Tetracycline, co-trimoxazole or streptomycin.

Vulvovaginitis in children

For details of this condition see Box 7.5.

Acute pelvic inflammatory disease

- Common problem with possible serious immediate complications, such as peritonitis and septicaemia and serious long-term sequelae of chronic pelvic inflammatory disease including infertility.
- Essential to diagnose accurately and to treat adequately and to examine sexual partner(s) and to treat them when necessary.

Aetiology

- Usually sexually transmitted, common organisms being *Chlamydia trachomatis, Neisseria gonorrhoeae* and *Mycoplasma hominis* (Box 7.6).

Box 7.5 Vulvovaginitis in children

Aetiology

- Poor hygiene
- Reaction to chemicals in soap, soap powder, bath salts etc.
- Vagina poorly protected in childhood
- May be due to sexual interference (exclude gonorrhoea and *Chlamydia*) or occasionally to presence of a foreign body
- Worms

Clinical features

- Soreness
- Discharge
- Dysuria

Examination and investigation

- General examination
- Examination of vulva, introitus and anus
- Take introital swab for culture
- Take swab from perianal region to look for worms
- Rectal examination to feel for foreign body in vagina, if indicated
- Occasionally examination of vagina under anaesthesia is required

Treatment

- Advice on hygiene and on avoiding possible chemical irritation
- Loose fitting cotton underwear
- Specific treatment for any demonstrable infection
- Removal of foreign body if present
- If no cause found and problem persists in spite of general measures, the application of a small amount of dienoestrol cream at night for 1–2 weeks will increase vaginal resistance to infection and may be helpful

Box 7.6 Organisms which may cause acute pelvic inflammatory disease

- *Chlamydia trachomatis* 50%
- *Neisseria gonorrhoeae* 10–15%
- *Mycoplasma hominis* 10–15%
- Anaerobic organisms such as *Bacteroides fragilis* and anaerobic streptococci
- Facultative anaerobes such as *Escherichia coli*
- β-Haemolytic streptococci
- *Actinomyces* spp.

- Commonest in young women and related to promiscuity of one or other partner.
- Much less commonly follows abortion or childbirth, or instrumentation such as dilatation and curettage, insertion of intrauterine contraceptive device (IUCD) or hysterosalpingography, major gynaecological surgery or appendicitis.

Clinical features

- Acute bilateral lower abdominal pain.
- Usually pyrexial and unwell; vomiting may occur.
- Vaginal discharge.
- On examination there is marked lower abdominal rebound tenderness and on vaginal examination there is marked adnexal tenderness and cervical excitation pain (pain on moving the cervix).

Investigations

- Cervical and urethral swabs including a cervical swab for *Chlamydia trachomatis.*
- Blood culture if patient severely ill.
- Clinical diagnosis may be uncertain and laparoscopy may be indicated. This will allow accurate diagnosis and swabs can be taken for culture.

Differential diagnosis

- Appendicitis.
- Ectopic pregnancy.
- Ovulation pain.

Box 7.7 Differential diagnosis

	Pain/tenderness	*Vomiting*	*Pyrexia*	*Bleeding*
Acute pelvic inflammatory disease	Both iliac fossae → hypochondria	±/+	⩾38°C	Sometimes irregular bleeding
Appendicitis	Umbilical → right iliac fossa	±/+	37–38°C	Normal cycle
Ectopic pregnancy	One or both iliac fossae Adnexal tenderness	–	⩽37°C	Usually amenorrhoea, then spotting
Ovulation pain	One → both iliac fossae	–	⩽37°C	Normal cycle; pain at mid-cycle
Torsion of ovarian cyst	One → both iliac fossae	+	⩽37°C	Normal cycle
Pyelonephritis	Unilateral loin pain → suprapubic region	±/+	⩾38°C	Normal cycle

- Torsion of an ovarian cyst or haemorrhage into a cyst.
- Pyelonephritis.

Treatment

- Bed rest and adequate analgesia.
- Adequate doses of appropriate antibiotics for at least 2 weeks – very important to eradicate infection completely. Tetracycline 500 mg 6-hourly for 14 days (or a cephalosporin) plus metronidazole 400 mg 12-hourly for 7 days. (Alcohol must not be taken during treatment with metronidazole.)
- If cultures reveal organisms not sensitive to the above treatment it must be changed appropriately.
- If patient's condition does not improve within 48 hours, the diagnosis must be reviewed and the treatment changed.
- No intercourse for at least 2 weeks after symptoms resolved and treatment finished.

Long-term sequelae

There is a 10–15% risk of permanent tubal damage after one episode of acute pelvic inflammatory disease, 25–30% risk after two episodes and a 50% risk after three episodes.

Chronic pelvic inflammatory disease

This is a common problem and can be very disabling.

Aetiology

- Usually follows one or more attacks of acute pelvic inflammatory disease especially if inadequately treated, but patient may be unaware that she has ever had pelvic inflammatory disease.
- Tuberculous salpingitis is rare in western Europe except in Asian immigrants.
- Actinomycosis is also rare but actinomycosis organisms may be found when an IUCD has been in place for a prolonged period of time.

Clinical features

Only one or two of these may be present and they may fluctuate in severity:

- Often unwell.
- Chronic lower abdominal pain and backache.
- Deep dyspareunia.
- Heavy periods.
- Dysmenorrhoea throughout period.

- Menstrual irregularity.
- Vaginal discharge.
- Infertility.
- Ectopic pregnancy may occur.
- On examination there may be reduced mobility of the uterus (often fixed retroversion) and there will be adnexal tenderness and sometimes adnexal masses.
- Very important not to assume that chronic pelvic pain is due to chronic pelvic inflammatory disease.

Differential diagnosis

- Endometriosis.
- Other causes of chronic pelvic pain (see Chapter 9).

Diagnosis

- Laparoscopy may be required to establish the diagnosis.

Treatment

- Superimposed acute infections should be treated with adequate antibiotic therapy.
- Intercourse should be avoided until symptoms have resolved.
- Surgical treatment may be required.

Chapter 8

Endometriosis

Endometriosis is a condition in which endometrium-like tissue is present in sites outside the uterus. The aetiology and pathophysiology of the condition are still poorly understood. Adenomyosis is a condition in which endometrium-like tissue is present in the myometrium. The aetiology and clinical features are different from those of endometriosis and this condition is considered later in this chapter.

Aetiology

- Endometriosis probably occurs most commonly as a result of retrograde menstruation along the fallopian tubes with spill into the peritoneal cavity followed by implantation of endometrial tissue onto the ovaries or peritoneal surfaces.
- Endometriosis may also arise by metaplasia of, for example, peritoneum.
- Lymphatic and haematogenous spread and direct implantation of endometrial tissue into a wound such as a laparotomy incision or episiotomy can occasionally occur.
- Following retrograde menstruation, some endometrial cells may implant; a localized inflammatory reaction may then occur followed in the peritoneum by typical puckering which may or may not be discoloured.
- Endometriotic deposits vary in size from microscopic to several centimetres in diameter.
- Marked adhesion formation may occur.
- It is not clear why some women develop clinical endometriosis and why others do not, nor why there is minimal or no adhesion formation in some women and gross adhesion formation in others.
- There appears to be some hereditary tendency to the development of endometriosis.

Sites

- The commonest sites for the development of endometriosis are the ovaries and pelvic peritoneum especially that lining the pouch of Douglas and covering the uterosacral ligaments (Figure 8.1). These are the areas most likely to be in contact with retrograde menstrual blood and tissue.
- Endometriotic (chocolate) cysts may occur on the ovaries and increase in size with each episode of menstruation. They are commonly bilateral.

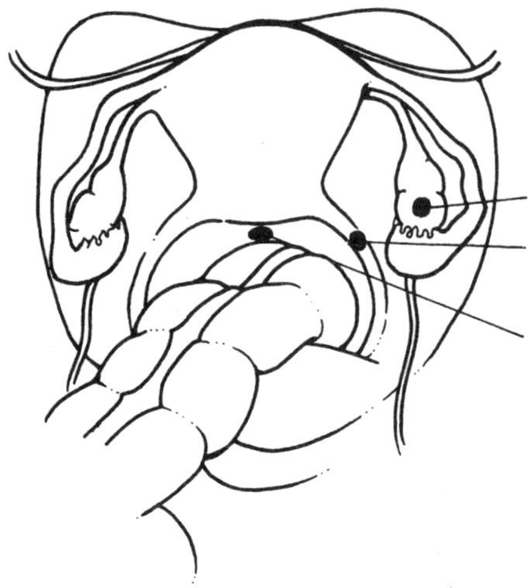

Figure 8.1 Common sites of endometriotic implants.

Symptoms

- Subfertility.
- Secondary dysmenorrhoea.
- Pelvic pain at other times in the cycle.
- Deep dyspareunia.
- Abnormal uterine bleeding.
- Pain on defaecation – uncommon.
- Urinary symptoms – uncommon.

General examination

- Usually no physical signs on general examination.
- Occasionally ovarian endometriotic (chocolate) cysts may be large enough to be palpable abdominally.

Vaginal examination

- Often no abnormality is detectable on vaginal examination.
- There may be palpable, often tender, nodules in the posterior fornix or uterosacral ligaments.
- The uterus may be fixed in a retroverted position by adhesions and there will then often be tenderness on palpation.
- The ovaries may be enlarged by palpable, usually fixed, chocolate cysts.

Diagnosis

Endometriosis can only be diagnosed by direct inspection at laparoscopy or laparotomy. Laparoscopy during menstruation may be helpful.

Differential diagnosis

The differential diagnosis will depend on predominant symptoms and signs but will usually include pelvic sepsis and, in the case of a pelvic swelling, other causes of a pelvic mass (see Chapter 19).

Classification

- Various classification systems have been developed to enable accurate description of findings and comparison between different modes of treatment to be made, but none is completely satisfactory.
- The revised American Fertility Society classification (*Fertility and Sterility* (1985) **43**, 351–352) is one that is commonly used at the present time.
- It is most important that a systematic search for endometriotic deposits is made at the time of laparoscopy and that a detailed diagrammatic and written description of the findings is made.

Endometriosis and subfertility

- Some 10% of infertile women have endometriosis as their only identifiable subfertility factor and some 30% of women with endometriosis are infertile.
- The more severe the manifestations of endometriosis, the more likely is the woman to be infertile but minimal endometriosis is a common finding in infertile women.
- The reason for the association between minimal endometriosis and infertility is not clear. Possible mechanisms that have been suggested include a direct toxic effect of abnormal constituents of peritoneal fluid, including prostaglandins, on sperm and tubal motility, fertilization and early growth of the embryo; abnormalities of the immune system; and ovulatory dysfunction. It has also been suggested that infertility predisposes to endometriosis.

Treatment of endometriosis

- Specific treatment for endometriosis should not be given until the diagnosis has been confirmed by laparoscopy or laparotomy.
- Recurrence of endometriosis after cessation of treatment is common and patients should be aware that medical treatment for endometriosis is seldom curative.
- Appropriate treatment will depend on the symptoms and operative findings.

- Treatment is not usually indicated for minimal asymptomatic endometriosis which can resolve spontaneously, but if the woman is requiring contraception a progestogenic combined pill would be a good choice if not otherwise contraindicated.

- *Persistent chocolate cysts* require surgical treatment, usually followed by medical treatment.

- *Infertility* – it is not clear how often mild or moderate endometriosis is the cause of infertility; there is no evidence that treatment of minimal endometriosis enhances fertility. Current medical treatment will render the woman infertile while she is being treated (usually for 6 or 9 months). Severe endometriosis usually warrants combined surgical and medical treatment in a woman complaining of infertility. Fertilization *in vitro* and gamete intrafallopian tube transfer (GIFT) have been used effectively in the management of infertility associated with endometriosis.

- *Pelvic pain* – mild pelvic discomfort may be reduced by a prostaglandin synthetase inhibitor such as mefenamic acid 500 mg three times daily or by a progestogenic combined contraceptive pill such as Ovran 30 or Eugynon 30 (ethinyl oestradiol 30 μg and levonorgestrel 250 μg) or Gynovlar (ethinyl oestradiol 50 μg and norethisterone 3 mg). Severe pelvic pain will require continuous hormonal therapy as described below. If severe pelvic pain in an older woman (over 40 years of age) is resistant to medical treatment, total hysterectomy and bilateral salpingo-oophorectomy should be considered; this may also be the treatment of choice in a younger women when fertility is no longer likely or desired.

Surgical treatment

- Ovarian cystectomy or intraovarian laser therapy is used in the treatment of chocolate cysts.
- Lysis of adhesions may be necessary, but adhesions are likely to recur.
- Small deposits of endometriosis can be treated by diathermy or laser ablation.

Medical treatment

- Steroid hormones are the main regulators of endometrial growth and function.
- Oestrogen stimulates endometrial growth and androgens cause atrophy of endometrial implants.
- The action of progestogens is less clear cut, but androgenic synthetic progestogens usually inhibit endometrial growth.
- Hormone treatment is effective if it either produces a low oestrogen environment or it is androgenic, or both.

Drugs used in the treatment of endometriosis

- Antiprostaglandins such as mefenamic acid 500 mg three times daily can be used for pelvic pain.

- Progestogenic combined oral contraceptives (such as Ovran and Gynovlar) can be used for contraception in mild and moderate endometriosis.
- Danazol 200–400 mg twice daily given continuously suppresses ovulation and causes amenorrhoea. Treatment is usually given for 6–9 months. Side-effects are common (Box 8.1).

Box 8.1 Danazol

- Isoxazole derivative of 17-α-ethinyl testosterone
- Suppresses ovulation and decreases oestrogen production
- Markedly decreases production of sex hormone-binding globulin (SHBG) and causes increase in free testosterone levels
- Causes atrophy of endometrial tissue by direct action as well as by above effects
- Lowers high-density lipoprotein (HDL) cholesterol levels
- Decreases thyroxine-binding globulin and total thyroxine levels; free thyroxine and TSH levels are unaffected
- Amenorrhoea should be aimed for and the dose increased up to 400 mg twice daily if necessary
- Weight gain, acne, hirsutism, oily skin and hot flushes are common and usually reversible side-effects; deepening of the voice may occur and may persist after stopping treatment
- Causes female pseudohermaphroditism in female fetuses and should therefore be started during a normal period to minimize the chance of administration during pregnancy; must be taken regularly and barrier contraception should be used

- Gestrinone 2.5 mg twice a week is a new 19-nortestosterone derivative (not yet available in this country) with efficacy and side-effects similar to those of danazol.
- LHRH agonists such as buserelin nasal spray (100 μg per nostril 4–6 times a day) or goserelin (subcutaneous depot implant once a month) reduce gonadotrophin stimulation of the ovaries thus producing reversible medical reduction of ovarian function and causing amenorrhoea. Hot flushes and other symptoms of oestrogen withdrawal are troublesome side-effects and long-term use is precluded by the risk of the development of osteoporosis.

Adenomyosis

Adenomyosis is a condition in which endometrium-like tissue (both glands and stroma) is present in the myometrium. The invasion of the myometrium is usually diffuse but may be in the form of adenomyomas which are spherical islands of endometrial and myometrial tissue, of up to a centimetre or more in diameter, intimately adherent to the surrounding myometrium.

Aetiology

- Cause unknown but it is accepted that the ectopic endometrium originates from the endometrial lining of the uterine cavity.

- Occurs mainly in multiparous women over 30 years of age.

Symptoms

- Increasingly severe dysmenorrhoea and pelvic discomfort.
- Menorrhagia.
- Deep dyspareunia.

Examination

- The uterus is enlarged, often irregular, and tender – not usually more than 10–12 weeks size unless fibroids are also present.

Diagnosis

- Can only be made with certainty by histological examination of the uterus.
- Diagnostic curettage will usually be required to exclude endometrial polyps, fibroid polyps and endometrial carcinoma.

Differential diagnosis

This depends on the particular symptoms and signs but includes fibroids, endometriosis, pelvic inflammatory disease, endometrial polyps and endometrial carcinoma (any of which may coexist with adenomyosis).

Treatment

- Mefenamic acid may alleviate menorrhagia and dysmenorrhoea to some extent.
- Hormonal treatment is not usually helpful, but norethisterone 5–10 mg a day from day 5 or 10 to day 25 of the menstrual cycle or continuous treatment with danazol 400–600 mg a day can be tried.
- If the symptoms are severe, hysterectomy is often the best option.

Chapter 9

Pelvic pain

Pelvic pain is a common presenting symptom which may be due to a variety of causes, both organic and non-organic (psychosomatic). It is important to establish the correct diagnosis and not to give inappropriate random treatment.

Pathophysiology of pelvic pain

- May originate in the genital, urinary or alimentary tracts, in the peritoneum, or in the musculoskeletal or central nervous systems.
- May be due to pressure on, or to inflammation, irritation, congestion, ischaemia or contractions of, the pelvic organs.
- Afferent pain neurones from intrapelvic structures travel via the dorsal nerve roots of the sacral nerves.
- Pain of pelvic origin is usually felt in the lower abdomen and back and may radiate down the thighs. The causes are listed in Box 9.1.

Management of patient complaining of chronic or recurring pelvic pain

It is important to exclude organic cause for the pain before assuming that it is not organic, but there may be pointers in the history and examination towards the likelihood that the pain is not organic in origin.

History

- Site of pain; any radiation.
- Type of pain – sharp or dull, constant or intermittent, colicky, burning or throbbing.
- Incapacitating or mainly a nuisance; interference with sleep.
- Duration and pattern of pain.
- What brings it on or aggravates it and what relieves it.
- Relationship to menstrual cycle.
- Past general history; any past history of similar pain.
- Obstetric and gynaecological history.
- Contraception.

Box 9.1 Common causes of pelvic pain

Acute pelvic pain (see Chapter 7)

Gynaecological
- Ovulation
- Acute salpingitis
- Ectopic pregnancy
- Haemorrhage into ovarian cyst
- Torsion of ovarian cyst or tumour
- Rupture of ovarian cyst

Other
- Cystitis
- Appendicitis
- Gastrointestinal disturbance
- Ureteric colic

Chronic pelvic pain

Gynaecological
- Primary dysmenorrhoea
- Secondary dysmenorrhoea
- Retrograde menstruation
- Ovulation pain
- Chronic pelvic sepsis
- Endometriosis
- Pelvic congestion
- Ovarian cyst or tumour
- Fibroids

Other
- Irritable bowel
- Constipation
- Psychosomatic
- Referred pain, e.g. from spine
- Diverticulitis
- Crohn's disease

- Psychosexual and social history.

Examination

- Full general and abdominal examination.
- Pelvic examination with particular reference to detecting what part of the examination, if any, causes discomfort.

Investigation

- The cause of chronic pelvic pain may be difficult to elucidate but there are likely to be pointers in the history and examination towards the diagnosis.
- Laparoscopy may be required to confirm or exclude a gynaecological cause for the pain, but is by no means invariably necessary. If, for example, it is thought that

recurrent pelvic pain is related to ovulation, sympathetic explanation and reassurance may be all that is necessary. If it is thought that the pain is due to the irritable bowel syndrome a trial of appropriate treatment should be instituted.

- It is very important to listen to the patient's views on the pain and to her concerns about it. Time taken at this stage is well spent and may save unnecessary investigation and treatment. She may be concerned that she has cancer and explanation and reassurance may be what is required rather than unnecessary investigation and treatment.

Non-organic psychosomatic pelvic pain

In many cases no organic cause is found for a complaint of pelvic pain.

- The patient is often polysymptomatic.
- There may be a social history of deprivation, marital disharmony or other stress.
- Psychosexual problems are common in this group but may be difficult to elicit.
- Abdominal and pelvic examination usually cause inconsistent and variable discomfort.
- A diagnosis of non-organic pelvic pain must not be made without careful exclusion of an organic basis for the pain.

Management

- Take a sympathetic history and perform a full examination with whatever investigations are indicated.
- Try to identify with the patient possible underlying stresses and their relationship to the pain. A calendar chart may be helpful.
- Endeavour to help the patient with sympathetic support, particularly if she is using the pain as a social crutch in which case she may not want to be cured.
- Important not to over-investigate or to overtreat, but equally important to identify and explain and/or treat the physical cause for the pain if there is one.

Chapter 10
Sexual dysfunction

The number of patients attending a doctor with acknowledged sexual dysfunction will depend on the cultural background of the patients and the perceived attitude of the doctor. Many patients present with gynaecological symptoms when their problems are psychosocial or psychosexual. If the doctor is not aware of this, patients may be inappropriately managed.

- Not all doctors have the time or ability to deal with sexual problems in depth but a sympathetic approach will help to resolve many problems. In other more complex cases, referral to a psychosexual counsellor will be appropriate.
- Psychosexual therapy requires good rapport between the therapist and the patient or couple and this may take time to achieve. Such therapy can be very time consuming and progress may be slow.
- An understanding of both male and female sexual function and dysfunction is necessary when providing counselling to the patient or to the couple.
- The gynaecologist must be aware of the concerns regarding sexual function of a patient who is advised to undergo surgical treatment – particularly vaginal surgery. Adequate explanation must be given to the patient who may not express her concerns directly.

Male sexual dysfunction

Normal male coital function requires arousal through mental, visual or tactile stimulation, erection (a parasympathetic function), penetration, ejaculation (a sympathetic function) and resolution.

Low sex drive and failure of arousal

- Congenitally diminished testicular function (as in Klinefelter's syndrome). Treatment with testosterone is likely to be beneficial if circulating levels are low.
- Psychiatric problems such as anxiety, depression and stress.
- Psychosocial and psychosexual problems due to marital disharmony or to latent or overt homosexuality. Counselling may be beneficial.
- Medications such as sedatives, tranquillizers and hypotensive drugs can reduce sex drive.

Impotence

- Congenital neurological problems such as spina bifida.
- Acquired neurological problems due to traumatic spinal tract damage or to a tumour.

- Psychiatric problems are commonly related to anxiety, depression or stress, or may follow an industrial or road traffic accident which leads to compensation orientated sexual dysfunction.
- Psychosocial and psychosexual maladjustment or malorientation.
- Medical disorders, e.g. diabetes, hyperprolactinaemia, myxoedema or liver failure.
- Drugs such as alcohol and psychotropic, anticholinergic and hypotensive medications. It is important to warn patients that sexual dysfunction is a possible side-effect of certain drugs.
- Psychoemotional problems following vasectomy.
- Disorders of the urogenital tract such as infection or Peyronie's disease. In Peyronie's disease a fibrous plaque develops between the fascia and the tunica albuginea of the corpora cavernosa causing angulation of the penis and pain on erection.

Management

- Appropriate counselling and treatment of medical problems or alteration of drug therapy.
- In a few patients surgical implantation of a penile prosthesis may be helpful.

Ejaculatory problems

- Congenital abnormalities such as hypospadias or phimosis.
- May be due to drugs which affect neurological control.
- *Premature ejaculation* is a common problem which can sometimes be treated effectively by squeezing the glans penis gently when the desire to ejaculate is felt, until the desire disappears. This process is repeated up to five times before ejaculation is allowed to occur. Treatment with clomipramine (25–75 mg a day) may also be helpful.
- *Ejaculatory incompetence* may occur with anxiety and stress.
- *Retrograde ejaculation* can occur, particularly after prostatectomy. Ejaculation with a full bladder may overcome the problem.

Female sexual dysfunction

Normal female sexual arousal occurs more through mental and tactile stimulation than by visual stimulation. During arousal lubricating secretions are produced. Intercourse can be pleasurable in the absence of orgasm which does not occur in all women.

Local problems

- An imperforate hymen or vaginal atresia will prevent penetration.
- Superficial or deep dyspareunia may lead to apareunia.

- Dyspareunia may be due to failure of arousal.
- Superficial dyspareunia may be due to infection such as candidiasis or trichomoniasis, or to atrophic vaginitis, or may occur following surgery such as an episiotomy or posterior repair.
- Deep dyspareunia may be due to pelvic inflammatory disease or endometriosis.

General problems

- Libido may be reduced by general debilitation or by oestrogen lack as in hypogonadotrophic hypogonadism, gonadal failure or hyperprolactinaemia.
- Drugs do not affect sexual function in women as much as in men, but libido may be reduced by oral contraception, phenothiazines and drugs of addiction in some women.
- Psychiatric problems such as anxiety, depression and psychosis commonly cause sexual dysfunction and require appropriate management and treatment.
- Psychosexual problems are a common cause and common result of marital disharmony. Management includes counselling of both partners often over a period of weeks or months.

History

- Obtaining a good history from a patient with sexual dysfunction is an art.
- A sympathetic unhurried, uncritical approach is essential.

Examination

- Thorough general and pelvic examination to exclude organic problems.
- The woman's response to pelvic examination may be a helpful indicator of the nature of the problem.

Management

- Depends on the problem.
- Local and general medical problems should be treated appropriately.
- Referral to a psychosexual counsellor or psychiatrist may be required.

Chapter 11

Subfertility

- Subfertility may be defined as lack of conception after one year of regular unprotected intercourse, as approximately 90% of normal couples in the reproductive age group conceive within a year of attempting conception (Box 11.1).

Box 11.1 Approximate conception rates with regular unprotected intercourse in normally fertile couples

1 month	25%
6 months	75%
9 months	85%
12 months	90%
24 months	95%

- May be primary (women not known to have ever conceived) or secondary (women who have had one or more proven pregnancies).
- It is a very common problem, because more than 10% of couples trying for a baby are involuntarily infertile.
- The pressures on many couples to have a baby are very strong and failure to achieve a pregnancy can cause great distress and may have profound psychosocial consequences.
- The benefits of thorough investigation include a probable explanation for the subfertility, a possible basis for treatment and a realistic prognosis.
- Ideally, the couple should attend together for at least the initial consultation so that their relationship can be assessed and the plan of investigation and possible treatment can be explained.
- The results of any previous investigations should be obtained to avoid duplication.
- In approximately 35% of couples a female factor is predominantly responsible, in 35% a male factor and in the remaining 30% of couples both female and male factors are responsible or no cause can be identified.
- The main causes of subfertility are defective ovulation (25%), defective spermatogenesis (25%), problems with gamete (sperm or egg) or fertilized ovum transport (25%), endometriosis and cervical mucus, immunological and sexual problems. In about 10% of cases no cause for the subfertility is found and, depending on the definition of unexplained infertility, a pregnancy will occur without treatment after several years of infertility in about 30% of these couples.
- Important to know when to stop investigation and treatment.

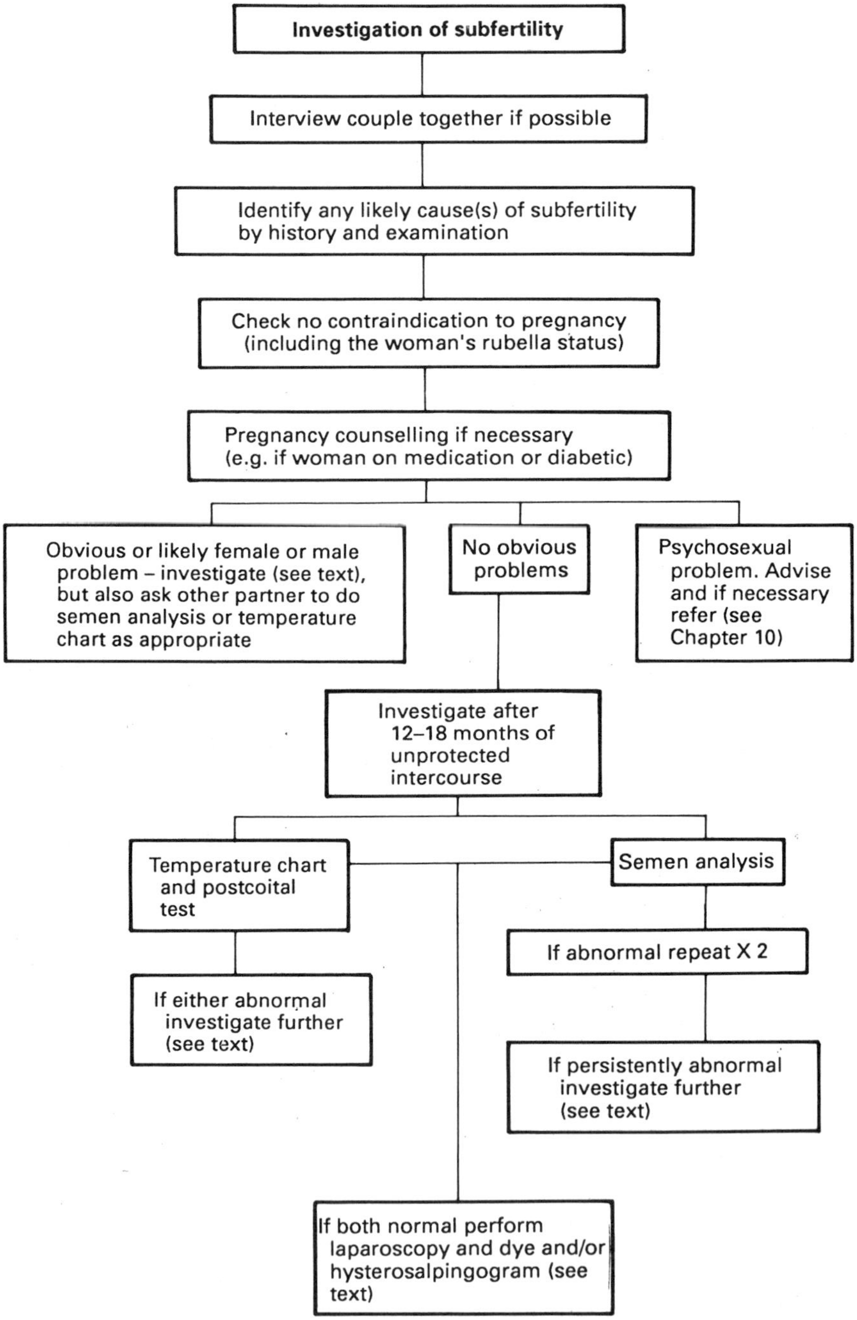

Figure 11.1 Investigation of subfertility.

Initial consultation

A general history is taken from each partner with regard to age, occupation, general wellbeing, previous contraception, any medication, past medical and surgical events, previous pregnancies and sexual function. The history and investigation of the male partner is discussed in detail in the next chapter and that of the female partner is discussed below.

Female partner

It is important to establish that the women is 'fit to be pregnant', i.e. that she has no disorder (such as hypertension, diabetes, a breast lump or an abnormal cervical smear) that should be investigated and treated before she becomes pregnant, that she is immune to rubella and that she is not taking any drugs that could have a deleterious effect on fetal development (such as warfarin, alcohol or nicotine). Appropriate prepregnancy counselling should be given at the initial consultation.

Specific points in history from female partner

General

- Age.
- Duration of subfertility.
- Details of pregnancies or lack of pregnancies with present or previous partners; time taken to conceive and any treatment required prior to conception.
- Previous forms of contraception and any complications arising from these, e.g. infection with IUCD.
- Previous investigations for subfertility.

Medical

- Age at menarche.
- Pattern of menstrual cycle since menarche.
- Date of last menstrual period.
- Any abnormal vaginal bleeding or discharge.
- Any history of sexually transmitted disease.
- Any other serious illnesses in the past or currently.
- Any drug treatment in the past or currently.
- Immunity or otherwise to rubella.

Surgical

- Any abdominal or other relevant surgery.

Social

- Occupation.
- Religion.
- Stress.
- Alcohol intake.
- Exposure to radiation, anaesthetics, chemicals.
- Drugs such as nicotine, marijuana or heroin.

Sexual

- Frequency and timing of intercourse (ideal frequency is 3–4 times a week or on alternate nights prior to and around the time of ovulation).
- Coital position.
- Problems with intercourse.
- Use of coital lubricants (these may be spermicidal).

Family

- Infertility.
- Genetic disorders.

Examination

- General examination including measurement of height and weight and blood pressure and examination of breasts.
- Vaginal examination including cervical smear if indicated.
- Urinalysis.

Investigations

If menstruating regularly and no obvious cause for infertility:

- Check rubella immunity.
- Basal body temperature chart and one midluteal progesterone 8 to 6 days before expected onset of a period (should be >30 nmol/l).
- Semen analysis (see Chapter 12).
- Correctly timed postcoital test.
- If above tests are satisfactory a test for tubal patency – usually laparoscopy with dye – should be performed after 12–18 months of regular unprotected intercourse.

If not menstruating regularly the appropriate investigations and treatment are described in Chapter 5.

Basal body temperature (BBT) chart

- There is a diurnal and activity-related variation in BBT. The temperature should be taken on waking and before rising in the morning.
- BBT charts are difficult to interpret in those doing night work. Even in those not doing night work they seldom look exactly like the example shown in fertility booklets and the patient should be told this and that it is difficult to be sure that ovulation has occurred except in retrospect as small temperature fluctuations are not uncommon.
- BBT is approximately 0.3°C or 0.5°F higher in the luteal phase because of the increased circulating progesterone level (see Figure 3.1). It is also increased by the exogenous administration of progesterone or progestogens.
- Luteal phase usually 10–14 days.
- BBT charts should not be used to time intercourse – once the temperature has definitely risen it is unlikely that conception will occur. The purpose of the BBT chart is to indicate in retrospect that a corpus luteum has been formed and that ovulation has probably occurred.
- If the pattern is consistent each month the BBT chart can be used to predict the day of ovulation in subsequent cycles to within 3 or 4 days.
- The best advice for timing intercourse is to have intercourse roughly every other night from days 8 to 16 in a regular 28-day cycle or from 4 days before to 3 days after the predicted temperature rise. It is important, however, that the couple are not mesmerized by the temperature chart.
- The BBT chart will give an early indication that pregnancy has occurred – if the temperature stays up for more than 16–18 days and menstruation does not occur it is likely that the woman is pregnant.
- Many women dislike doing BBT charts and if three cycles are normal they should be encouraged to stop if they want to.
- If the BBT chart is abnormal further investigation in the form of serial pelvic ultrasound scans during one cycle and/or serial progesterone estimations in the luteal phase should be performed.

Postcoital test

- Timing is very important. It is only positive when cervical mucus is made receptive by high preovulatory oestrogen levels on day 11 to 14 of a 28-day cycle.
- Demoralizing for the patient, her partner and the doctor if she is tested on the wrong day of the cycle with a consequent negative result.
- Couple should have intercourse as usual on the night before the test. The sperms should remain active in the mucus for at least 18 hours and so the woman can be examined in a morning or afternoon clinic.

Box 11.2 Technique of postcoital test

- Time by previous BBT records or choose day 12 or 13 of cycle if normally 28 days
- If difficult to time by previous BBT, can be timed by ovulation predictor kit which detects LH surge in the urine
- Normal intercourse the night before the examination
- No douching or bathing
- Insert unlubricated vaginal speculum to expose the cervix and aspirate the mucus with a quill or plastic capillary tube
- The external os should be gaping at time of ovulation
- Examine mucus immediately under the microscope
- The mucus should be clear and stretchable and there should be more than three to five motile sperms moving purposefully per high power field.

Box 11.3 Negative postcoital test

Poor quality mucus, i.e. scanty and/or cellular

- Wrong time in cycle
- Infection
- Poor cervical mucus production

No sperms at all

- Wrong time in cycle
- Apareunia
- Retrograde ejaculation
- Azoospermia

Few, poorly moving or dead sperms

- Wrong time in cycle
- Infection
- Poor quality mucus
- Poor quality sperms
- Antisperm antibodies in one or other partner

Further investigation

- Semen analysis if not already performed
- Check sexual history
- Check timing in cycle and repeat postcoital test at appropriate time
- Cervical mucus penetration (crossed hostility) test (Box 11.4) and Kibrick (blood) test for antisperm antibodies in both partners

Box 11.4 Crossed hostility test

Normal 'donor' sperms are placed on a slide next to the patient's ovulatory cervical mucus stretched along the line of its strands and some of the partner's sperms are placed on a slide with normal 'donor' ovulatory cervical mucus. The rate of invasion and activity of the sperms are observed under the microscope.

Tubal patency tests

These are invasive and should not usually be undertaken until it has been shown that ovulation and spermatogenesis are occurring, and the couple have been trying for a baby for at least a year.

- *Tubal insufflation* – carbon dioxide is delivered using a special apparatus via cannula placed in the cervix and the pressure is recorded. This technique is seldom used now as it is an inefficient way of confirming normality or diagnosing pathology and cannot distinguish between unilateral and bilateral tubal patency. It can, however, be used as an initial outpatient screening test.
- *Hysterosalpingography* – radiopaque dye is introduced via a cannula placed in the cervix and screening is performed and appropriate X-ray pictures are taken (Figures 11.2 and 11.3). It is a useful technique for demonstrating intrauterine and intratubal pathology and is a useful alternative to laparoscopy when this is contraindicated. Many patients find the procedure uncomfortable and it is very important that they should be told what to expect. The technique for hysterosalpingography is given in Box 11.5.

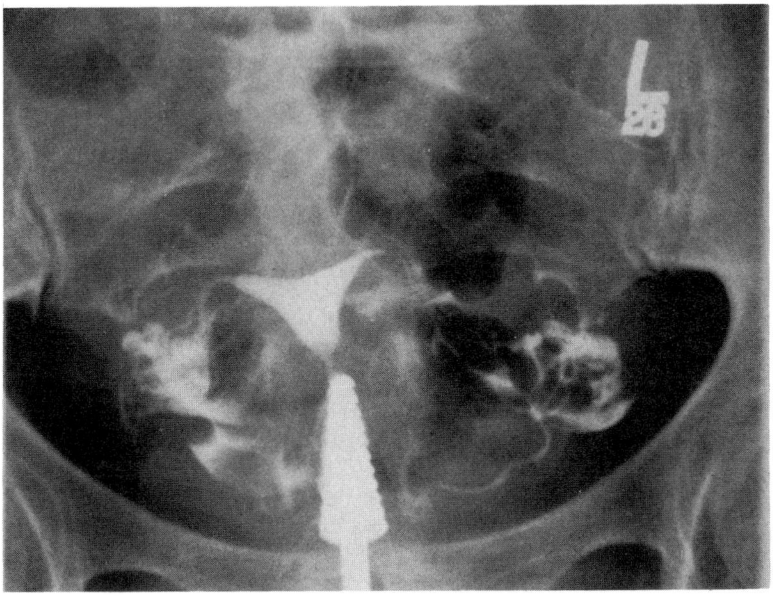

Figure 11.2 Normal hysterosalpingogram.

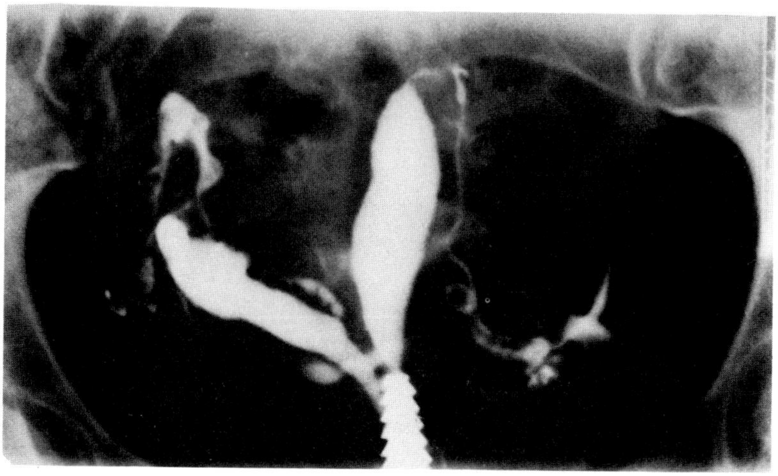

Figure 11.3 Double uterus.

Box 11.5 Technique of hysterosalpingography

- Perform in follicular phase of cycle to ensure that the patient is not pregnant
- Make sure that she is not allergic to iodine and that she understands the procedure and that it will be uncomfortable
- Give prophylactic antiprostaglandin (e.g. mefenamic acid 500 mg) if considered necessary
- Ask her to empty her bladder and then to lie supine on the couch
- Elevate the legs using lithotomy poles if necessary and clean the vulva and vagina with antiseptic
- Perform a bimanual examination to exclude unexpected pathology or pregnancy
- Gently insert a bivalve speculum and grasp cervix with tenaculum after warning patient about what is going to happen
- Fill the syringe and then the cannula with radiopaque dye and insert into cervical canal
- When the radiologist is ready introduce the dye slowly into the uterine cavity, tubes and peritoneal cavity watching what is happening on the screen; move the cervix gently if necessary with the tenaculum to improve the angle of the uterus and to check mobility
- Ask the radiologist to take two or three appropriate pictures
- When the procedure is finished remove the instruments and allow the patient to rest for as long as necessary

- *Laparoscopy with dye* – visualization of the pelvic organs must be performed before subfertility can be said to be unexplained. Abnormalities of the tubes, peritubal adhesions and endometriosis will commonly be found.
- *Hysteroscopy* can be performed at the same time. It is useful in the elucidation of intrauterine abnormalities.

Uterine causes of infertility

- Assessed by hysterosalpingography and/or by hysteroscopy.
- *Fibroids* – these are very common but are seldom the cause of infertility. Many women with fibroids have straightforward pregnancies and fibroids are usually best left alone in women who are trying to become pregnant unless they are symptomatic or there is a strong likelihood that they are the cause of infertility. Fibroid polyps and those blocking the intramural portions of both tubes can clearly cause infertility and should be treated surgically. Submucous fibroids may also cause infertility.
- *Uterine malformations* – these seldom cause infertility. Many women with uterine malformations have successful pregnancies.
- *Asherman's syndrome* – traumatic intrauterine adhesions (see Chapter 5).

Treatment of female infertility

The investigation and treatment of amenorrhoea and oligomenorrhoea are discussed in Chapter 5.

Long cycles (long follicular phase)

Some women have ovulatory cycles with a long follicular phase and may have a cycle length of up to 35–42 days; ovulation then only occurs 9 or 10 times a year. Treatment with clomiphene citrate 50 mg a day for 3 days from the third day of the cycle will often shorten the follicular phase to a normal length and cause ovulation to occur more frequently and more predictably.

Short luteal phase or inadequate luteal progesterone level

- These will be diagnosed from the temperature chart and the luteal progesterone level (measured 8–6 days before the next period).
- First line treatment is with clomiphene citrate 50 mg a day for 3–5 days from the third day of cycle, as an inadequate luteal phase is often associated with an inadequate follicular phase. If this treatment is unsuccessful exclusion of endocrine abnormalities such as hyperprolactinaemia and thyroid disorders, as well as ultrasound evaluation of ovarian function during the cycle, is indicated.

Treatment of poor quality cervical mucus

- Treat infection if present.
- Preovulatory low dose oral oestrogen.
- Follicular phase menopausal gonadotrophin administration to increase endogenous oestrogen level.
- Intrauterine or pouch of Douglas insemination with prepared sperms.

- Assisted conception using GIFT or *in vitro* fertilization (see below).

Tubal problems

- Tubal surgery for problems due to past tubal infection has a low success rate because, even if tubal patency can be restored, the epithelium is often severely damaged and therefore normal transport of the gametes and fertilized ovum is impaired. The overall success rate is approximately 10–20%, but will depend very much on the extent of damage in a particular case. It is only indicated when other causes of infertility have been excluded. For contraindications to surgery see Box 11.6.
- Success will be most likely when there are peritubal adhesions, but the tubes themselves are normal, and least likely where the tubes are damaged and distorted. The patient must be warned about the subsequent increased risk of an ectopic pregnancy.
- Reversal of sterilization has a very good success rate if the tubes are otherwise normal and if only a small segment of the tube has been damaged by surgery. Thus the success rate of reversal of clip sterilization is approximately 80% but there is little chance of successful reversal following diathermy sterilization.

Box 11.6 Contraindications to tubal surgery

- Contraindications to pregnancy
- Refractory anovulation
- Poor semen analysis
- Refractory poor postcoital test
- Severe tubal damage

Endometriosis

- The management of this condition is discussed in Chapter 8.

Sexual problems

- Give appropriate advice or refer for psychosexual counselling if necessary (see Chapter 10).

Unexplained infertility

The definition of unexplained infertility will differ from one centre to another and becomes more complex as new techniques of investigation are developed.

Basic criteria

- Normal history and normal examination of both partners.

- A history of 2 or more years of involuntary infertility with regular intercourse.
- Cycle length less than 42 days with normal luteal phase determined by temperature chart and midluteal progesterone level.
- Normal semen quality as judged by examination of two ejaculates (volume 2–6 ml; count ⩾ 20 million/ml; progressive motility ⩾ 50% at 1–2 hours; abnormal forms < 30%; MAR test negative).
- Normal postcoital test.
- Normal laparoscopic findings with passage of dye, with no evidence of tubal damage, adhesions or endometriosis.

Additional criteria

- Normal ovarian function as determined by ultrasound monitoring of one cycle.
- Normal hysterosalpingogram.
- A further semen specimen subjected to further evaluation as available, e.g. hamster oocyte penetration test.

In vitro fertilization and other related techniques

Major advances are occurring in the treatment of subfertility using a combination of induction of multiple ovulation and oocyte retrieval and replacement either before or after fertilization.

In vitro fertilization

- This was the first such technique to be described. In most centres multiple folliculogenesis is induced, using a combination of clomiphene and human menopausal gonadotrophin, and monitored by ovarian ultrasound. Human chorionic gonadotrophin is administered when there are an appropriate number of follicles ⩾ 18 mm.
- Ovum retrieval is performed by laparoscopy or ultrasound directed needle aspiration 36 hours later, before ovulation occurs. The partner's fresh washed sperms are incubated with the oocytes. If fertilization occurs up to three or occasionally four fertilized ova at the 4–8 cell stage are placed in the uterine cavity 48–72 hours later, via a fine flexible tube passed through the cervix.
- Any spare fertilized ova can be frozen and replaced at a later date.
- The pregnancy rate using this technique is of the order of 10–20% if fertilization occurs.
- Unfortunately, the miscarriage rate is approximately 25% and there is a risk of ectopic pregnancy.
- The technique has been used with success in cases of tubal damage, endometriosis, luteinized unruptured follicle syndrome, cervical mucus problems, oligoasthenospermia, antisperm antibodies and unexplained infertility.

- The take home baby rate is approximately 10% per procedure, depending on the indication for treatment and the age of the patient.

Gamete intrafallopian tube transfer (GIFT)

- Multiple folliculogenesis is induced using clomiphene and human menopausal gonadotrophin, and human chorionic gonadotrophin is administered when there are an appropriate number of follicles $\geqslant 18$ mm.
- Laparoscopic ovum retrieval is performed 36 hours later; one or two mature ova and approximately 50 000 fresh washed sperm are introduced into each fallopian tube to a depth of about 2 cm via the fimbrial end of the tube using a fine flexible cannula.
- Any spare ova can be fertilized and frozen and replaced at a later date.
- The pregnancy rate using this technique is of the order of 30–35%.
- Unfortunately, the miscarriage rate is of the order of 20%.
- The take home baby rate is approximately 20% per procedure depending on the indication for treatment and the age of the patient.

Chapter 12
Male subfertility

Incidence

In approximately 50% of cases, subfertility is wholly or partly due to a male factor.

Normal testicular function

- Testicular function is regulated by luteinizing hormone (LH) and follicle stimulating hormone (FSH) produced by the pituitary.
- LH stimulates synthesis and secretion of testosterone (T) by Leydig cells; its effect is enhanced by FSH. Increasing T levels inhibit LH secretion.
- FSH with T stimulates spermatogenesis in the seminiferous tubules. FSH production is decreased by inhibin produced by the Sertoli cells of the testes.
- Production of mature sperms takes nearly 3 months so a poor semen analysis may be due to adverse factors – such as febrile illness – occurring several weeks previously.

Causes of male subfertility

Congenital abnormality of hypothalmic–pituitary–testicular–ejaculatory axis

- Kallman's syndrome – congenital lack of LHRH production. There will be no pubertal development and there is often associated anosmia.
- Sex chromosome abnormalities, such as Klinefelter's syndrome – XXY – or mosaic. Typically eunuchoid body habitus, small, firm testes and azoospermia or severe oligospermia. FSH is elevated.
- Germ cell aplasia with normal sex chromosomes. Azoospermia, elevated FSH, normal testosterone.
- Cryptorchidism – even if cryptorchid testes are brought down early in childhood they usually fail to function normally.
- Congenital aplasia of vasa deferentia.
- Anatomical abnormalities of penis such as hypospadias.

Acquired abnormality of the hypothalamic–pituitary–testicular–ejaculatory axis

- Hypothalamic or pituitary tumours or damage.

- Acquired testicular malfunction may be due to generalized disease, local trauma or infection (such as mumps), endocrine abnormalities, drugs, heat, irradiation or immunological abnormalities, but is commonly idiopathic.
- Acquired blockage of the epididymis or vas deferens may be caused by infection, or surgery such as vasectomy or herniorrhaphy.
- Problems with ejaculation may be due to generalized disease (such as diabetes, neurological disorders or vascular insufficiency), drugs or alcohol, or may be psychological in origin (see Chapter 10).

Specific points in history from male partner

General

- Age.
- Duration of subfertility.
- Pregnancies or lack of pregnancies with previous partners.

Medical

- Cryptorchidism.
- Timing of puberty.
- Testicular disease or trauma.
- Mumps orchitis.
- Any serious illness in the past or currently.
- Any drug treatment particularly benzodiazepines, nitrofurantoin, sulphasalazine.
- Chemotherapy or radiotherapy.
- Any illness or drugs in last 3 months that might affect spermatogenesis.

Surgical

- Orchidopexy.
- Herniorrhaphy.
- Vasectomy.
- Testicular surgery.

Social

- Occupation.
- Exposure of testes to excessive heat – tight pants, hot working environment, sauna.
- Stress.
- Alcohol intake.

- Exposure to radiation or chemicals.
- Drugs such as nicotine, marijuana or heroin.

Sexual

- Frequency and timing of intercourse.
- Problems with intercourse.
- Coital position.
- Ensure that erection, penetration, ejaculation and seminal emission occur.
- Use of coital lubricants.

Family

- Infertility.
- Genetic disorders.

Examination of male partner

- Height and weight.
- Body habitus.
- Ability to smell.
- Visual fields.
- Hair distribution.
- Breasts – gynaecomastia, galactorrhoea.
- External genitalia – feel testicular consistency and assess size. Maximum length should be more than 3 cm and volume (assessed with orchidometer, Figure 12.1) more than 15 ml.

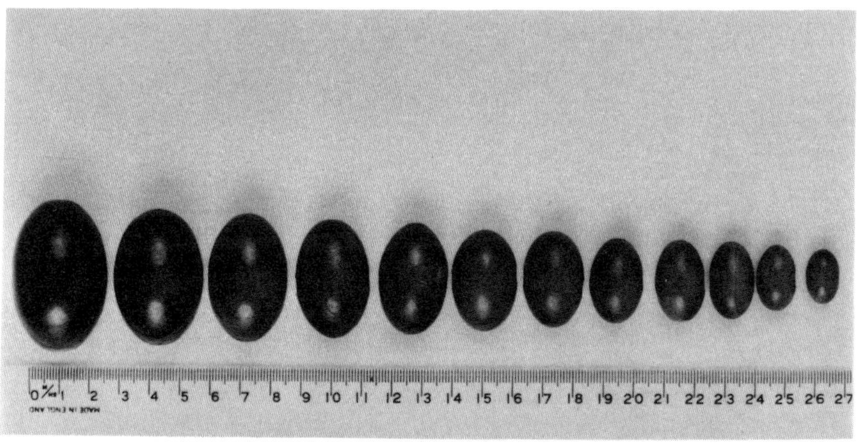

Figure 12.1 Orchidometer.

- Examine for varicocele (present in 20% of fertile and infertile men, usually on the left side). Examine standing up and during Valsalva manoeuvre. Arrange Doppler studies if necessary.
- Check epididymis and spermatic cord for nodularity.
- Rectal examination to check prostate and seminal vesicles. Massage to check secretions.

Investigation

- Semen analysis including MAR test (see below).
- FSH and testosterone if azoospermic or oligoasthenospermic.
- Karyotype if indicated.
- Urethral swab for sexually transmitted infection if likely from the history or examination.
- Testicular biopsy is rarely indicated.
- Kibrick test – blood test for antisperm antibodies – if MAR test positive.

Semen analysis

Although ideally both the man and the woman should be seen together very often the woman comes on her own, at least initially. A semen sample should be requested and if abnormal repeated at least twice with a gap of a few weeks.

Box 12.1 Semen analysis

- Specimen preferably produced after 3 days abstinence – consistent interval allows comparison of samples
- Collect ejaculate produced by masturbation (not withdrawal) into a wide-mouthed sterile container (not a condom)
- Protect specimen from temperature fluctuations and bring to laboratory within 1–2 hours of ejaculation
- Liquefaction should occur within 20 minutes of ejaculation
- The specimen must be thoroughly mixed before it is examined under the microscope

Normal parameters

Volume	2–6 ml
Density	20–200 million/ml
Motility	More than 50% progressively motile 1–2 hours after ejaculation; little or no agglutination
Morphology	More than 70% normal; no leucocytes

- *If semen analysis abnormal* check that instructions were adhered to and obtain two further specimens at least 2–4 weeks apart. If these are abnormal take a full history from the male partner and examine him or refer him to an andrologist.

- *Low volume* may be due to spillage, frequent ejaculation, retrograde ejaculation (check a centrifuged post-ejaculation urine specimen for sperms), aplasia of vasa deferentia, abnormality of prostate or seminal vesicles (check fructose) or to no obvious cause.
- *Azoospermia* (complete absence of sperms from ejaculate) may be due to testicular failure, blockage of seminiferous ducts (obstructive azoospermia), retrograde ejaculation or hypothalamic or pituitary disease.
- *Oligospermia* may be due to stress, drugs (including nicotine and alcohol), environmental or endocrine abnormalities, but is commonly idiopathic.
- *Poor motility* may be due to collection in a condom containing spermicide, delay in examining the specimen, chilling of the specimen, infection or immunological problems or dead sperms (necrospermia), but is commonly idiopathic.
- *Agglutination* of sperms may be due to infection or immunological problems.
- *The presence of leucocytes* may indicate inflammation of the prostate or seminal vesicles and examination of the man and of his prostatic secretions should be performed.

Other tests on semen

- *Fructose* – produced by seminal vesicles and absent when seminal vesicles absent (e.g. in aplasia of vasa deferentia); reduced when seminal vesicles inflamed.
- *MAR (mixed erythrocyte spermatozoal antiglobulin reaction) test* – erythrocytes sensitized with anti-IgG or -IgA antibody are mixed with the semen. If agglutination occurs it indicates that antisperm antibodies are present.
- *Kremer test* measures ability of sperms to penetrate a column of mucus in a capillary tube. The distance penetrated, the density of penetration and the motility of the sperms at a particular level in the tube are noted at specific times.
- *Zona free hamster oocyte penetration test* – exact significance of test not yet clear but reduced penetration correlates with inability to fertilize human ova.

Treatment of male subfertility

- The treatment of male subfertility is often unrewarding but in a few cases specific treatment is available.
- Kallman's syndrome – prolonged treatment with pulsatile LHRH or menopausal gonadotrophins and HCG.
- Alteration of alcohol intake or drug treatment may be beneficial.
- Azoospermia due to obstruction merits exploration if the testes are of normal size and the FSH level is normal.
- Oligospermia and poor motility may sometimes be improved by ensuring environmental temperature not too high and by wearing loose underpants. Cold scrotal sponging may be beneficial. If a varicocele is present ligation should be considered but its value is debatable.

- Antisperm antibodies in the male are associated with a poor prognosis. High dose corticosteroid treatment has been tried but is associated with severe side-effects such as aseptic necrosis of the head of the femur, and has largely been abandoned; lower dose corticosteroid treatment of the male during the follicular phase of the female partner's cycle and management by intrauterine insemination are being evaluated.
- Vasectomy reversal results in patency in more than 50% of cases, but often fertility is not restored because of the development of antisperm antibodies. (Approximately 10–20% pregnancy rate in 2 years following vasectomy reversal.)
- Hypospadias may be improved surgically.
- Erectile failure may require psychosexual counselling or surgical treatment (see Chapter 10).
- Ejaculatory problems may be resolved by treatment of the cause or occasionally by artificial insemination of the husband's semen if ejaculation occurs with masturbation.
- Retrograde ejaculation may be overcome by ejaculating with a full bladder or viable sperms may be recovered from a centrifuged post-ejaculatory urine specimen and used for artificial insemination (the urine must be rendered alkaline prior to ejaculation).

Artificial insemination with husband's semen (AIH)

Indications

- Unable to ejaculate into vagina but able to ejaculate by masturbation.
- Severe hypospadias or other anatomical abnormality.
- Refractory premature ejaculation.
- Retrograde ejaculation (if ejaculation with full bladder fails).
- Idiopathic low volume semen specimen with negative postcoital test.
- High volume semen specimen – split the ejaculate and artificially inseminate the fraction with the most normal motile sperms (usually the first fraction).
- Semen may be frozen for insemination at a later date from men about to have treatment with chemotherapy or radiotherapy for, for example, testicular tumours or Hodgkin's disease.

Technique of intracervical insemination

- Only applicable at time of ovulation and so basal body temperature/mucus chart should be kept or ovulation predictor kit or ultrasound can be used to help time insemination.
- On day chosen for insemination collect semen obtained by masturbation in sterile container.
- Keep semen at body temperature.

- Inseminate semen into external cervical os within 2 hours of ejaculation.
- Technique can be learnt by male partner in some cases to allow insemination at home.

Intrauterine insemination

- Semen sample taken to laboratory within 1–2 hours of ejaculation.
- Semen washed and concentrated by swim-up technique in buffer solution and is then instilled into uterine cavity via fine catheter.

Artificial insemination with donor semen (AID)

- This may be indicated if the male partner has azoospermia or severe oligospermia or other untreatable forms of infertility, or in some hereditary disorders.
- Very careful thought must be given by the couple before choosing to undergo treatment by AID and in-depth counselling by the clinician and a trained counsellor is essential. The couple must be aware of the possible psychological consequences of this form of treatment and that there is no guarantee in an AID pregnancy (as in any other pregnancy) that the child will be normal. They must also be aware of the legal situation and of the possible effects on the child of finding out that he/she was conceived by AID.
- Donors must be very carefully screened for hereditary and sexually transmitted disease (including AIDS and hepatitis B) and strict confidentiality is essential. The semen is collected and frozen. The donor is retested for AIDS 3 months later and if negative the frozen semen can be used.
- An attempt must be made to match the physical characteristics of the donor with those of the husband.
- Correct timing of insemination is essential.
- Ninety per cent of pregnancies that will occur, occur within 6–12 months.
- The overall success rate with fresh semen is about 70% and with frozen semen is about 50%.

Box 12.2 Sequence of events in AID

- *First session* – husband and wife interviewed and full discussion undertaken with them of all relevant points. Reservations and fears must be aired. Examination and investigations undertaken if indicated. Literature on AID is provided to be read at leisure. Basal body temperature chart commenced
- *Second session* – further full discussion. Obtain results of any tests and investigations and look at temperature chart. Arrange for social worker to visit if thought necessary
- *Third session* – decide whether treatment should be commenced. Complete consent form and arrange a starting date

Chapter 13

Bleeding in early pregnancy, miscarriage, ectopic pregnancy and hydatidiform mole

Bleeding in early pregnancy

Bleeding in early pregnancy is a common problem and very worrying for the woman concerned. It may settle with no long-term sequelae, or it may herald a miscarriage or another pregnancy complication, or be due to a problem unrelated to the pregnancy (Box 13.1). Sympathetic counselling is of the utmost importance whatever the diagnosis.

Box 13.1 Causes of bleeding in early pregnancy

- Threatened abortion
- Complete abortion
- Incomplete abortion
- Missed abortion
- Septic abortion
- Ectopic pregnancy
- Hydatidiform mole/choriocarcinoma
- Cervical ectropion
- Cervical polyp
- Cervical carcinoma

General approach

- Confirm that the woman is in fact pregnant by history and examination, and by pregnancy test or additional investigations such as ultrasound and βHCG if necessary.
- If a continuing intrauterine pregnancy is confirmed by ultrasound, reassure the women that the risk of miscarriage is less than 5% and that if the pregnancy does continue there is no increased risk of fetal abnormality.
- If the pregnancy is not continuing the woman will usually be very distressed. A miscarriage is often a devastating experience for the woman or couple concerned (see later in chapter).

Miscarriage/abortion

These words are synonymous but the word miscarriage should be used when possible for a spontaneous miscarriage as to many women 'abortion' implies induced abortion. The current definition is the expulsion of the products of conception before week 28 of gestation but this definition needs to be changed as many healthy surviving babies have been born before 28 weeks' gestation (i.e. less than 26 weeks after conception). The World Health Organisation definition is the expulsion of a fetus weighing 500 g or less or before 22 weeks' gestation.

Miscarriage

Spontaneous miscarriage occurs in about 15% of clinically confirmed pregnancies – usually in the first 3 months. Many more miscarriages occur before pregnancy is confirmed.

Box 13.2 Aetiology of miscarriage

- Commonest cause of first trimester miscarriage is abnormality of the embryo or chorion which is severe enough to cause death of the embryo. An embryonic chromosomal abnormality has been found in 50% of first trimester miscarriages in some studies – the most common abnormalities being trisomy, XO and triploidy
- Increased incidence with increasing maternal age
- Second trimester miscarriages are less common but more likely to have an identifiable cause such as cervical incompetence, fetal abnormality, multiple pregnancy, placental abruption, uterine anomaly, or maternal disorders such as infection, antibodies, diabetes, hypertension, renal disease etc. (see below)

Threatened miscarriage

- Bleeding from the uterus in the first (or much less commonly second) trimester.
- A very common problem.
- Sometimes lower abdominal discomfort but no actual pain.
- Uterus compatible in size with dates and cervical os closed.
- If the fetal heart is seen to be beating on ultrasound (should be possible with a normal pregnancy from 8 weeks' gestation onwards) the risk of miscarriage is less than 5%.
- If the fetus is alive advise rest and no intercourse for two weeks. Drug therapy is not helpful. In particular, progestogens are of no proven value and might be harmful; they can certainly prolong the time to spontaneous miscarriage after a fetus has died, causing a missed abortion. Some progestogens cause masculinization of a female fetus.
- Reassure the patient that bleeding does not increase the likelihood of fetal abnormality if miscarriage does not ensue.

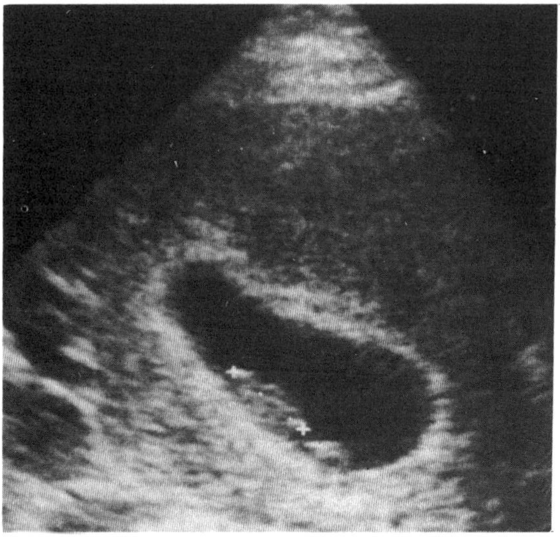

Figure 13.1 Eight-week embryo on ultrasound.

- Ask the patient to save any clots or tissue that are passed.
- If bleeding becomes heavier and painful contractions occur, miscarriage is likely. The patient may require admission to hospital. Give analgesics as necessary, having excluded the possibility of an ectopic pregnancy.

Complete abortion

- Implies that all the products of conception have been expelled.
- On vaginal examination the uterus is bulky but small for dates, the cervical os is closed and the bleeding is not heavy and stops after a few days.
- An ultrasound scan will show an empty uterine cavity.
- Anti-D immunoglobulin (250 units) should be given within 72 hours if the woman is rhesus negative.

Incomplete abortion (Figure 13.2)

- Many spontaneous miscarriages are incomplete, particularly between 8 and 14 weeks' gestation.
- Retention of placental tissue leads to continued bleeding and risk of infection.
- Expelled placental tissue may be identified; the uterus will be enlarged and there may be retained tissue in the cervical os.
- If bleeding heavily give ergometrine 0.25 mg slowly intravenously and repeat if necessary.
- Resuscitate if necessary. Take blood for full blood count, group and save serum.
- Products in the os may increase shock and can be removed using a speculum and sponge-holding forceps if necessary.

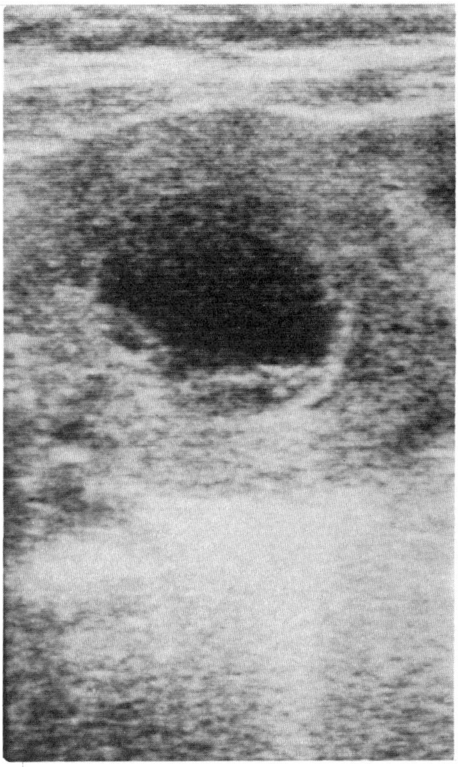

Figure 13.2 Incomplete abortion on ultrasound. (Courtesy of Dr Peter Twining)

- If the diagnosis is uncertain ultrasound examination will show whether the uterus is empty or not.
- Take patient to theatre and perform evacuation of retained products of conception (ERPC; Box 13.3).

Box 13.3 Evacuation of retained products of conception

- Full blood count, group and save serum
- General or spinal anaesthesia
- Sterile precautions – clean and drape patient
- Catheterization seldom necessary
- Assess the size of the uterus and explore the cavity digitally if possible
- Give 5 units syntocinon or ergometrine 0.25 mg slowly intravenously
- Use suction evacuation or sponge-holding forceps, and a blunt curette if necessary, to complete evacuation; be very careful to avoid excessive curettage
- Monitor pulse and blood pressure on return to ward
- Give 250 units anti-D immunoglobulin if woman is rhesus negative

Missed abortion

- Implies that the fetus has died but that miscarriage has not occurred.
- The woman will notice cessation of pregnancy symptoms; the uterus will be small for dates, a brown vaginal loss will occur and the pregnancy test will eventually become negative – this may take several days.
- Confirm the diagnosis with ultrasound. This will show no fetal heart activity and a collapsed, usually empty sac. Remember that a small-for-dates uterus with a small sac may just be due to wrong dates. If any doubt repeat the scan 1 week later.
- Once the diagnosis is certain many women will prefer elective evacuation rather than spontaneous miscarriage.
- Check clotting factors because of risk of disseminated intravascular coagulation with a missed abortion; the risk of this complication increases with time and gestational age.
- Group and save serum.
- Evacuate the uterus. If 12 weeks size or less, by suction evacuation. If larger, by administration of a prostaglandin pessary and then intravenous syntocinon if necessary.

Septic abortion

- Incomplete abortion with intrauterine infection.
- Much less common in the UK since the Abortion Act of 1967. Most severe cases of septic abortion before that were due to interference.
- The woman presents with an incomplete abortion and fever. She may be shocked due to septicaemia. There will be tachycardia, lower abdominal pain, pelvic tenderness and purulent vaginal discharge. There may be no fever with Gram-negative septicaemia (Box 13.4).
- Take cervical swab for urgent microscopy and culture and take blood for blood culture, full blood count, group and save serum.
- Resuscitation and antibiotic therapy must precede surgical evacuation of the uterus. Amoxycillin 500 mg (or a cephalosporin) and metronidazole 400 mg can be commenced while awaiting bacteriology results.
- Microscopy may reveal *Clostridium perfringens* (*welchii*) in which case penicillin is the treatment of choice.
- Watch for renal failure and haemoglobinuria (in clostridial infection) – maintain a fluid chart.
- Continue appropriate antibiotic therapy for at least a week after temperature settles to minimize chance of long-term sequelae such as chronic salpingitis.

Emotional effects of miscarriage

- The loss of even a very early pregnancy is usually a deeply distressing event for the woman and her partner.

- Many emotions will come to the surface at different times in the days and weeks following miscarriage. These include fear of the process of miscarriage and about the future, profound disappointment, grief, anger, self-pity, feelings of inadequacy, failure and helplessness, guilt, jealousy of those who have got children, overwhelming sadness and sometimes prolonged depression. It is important to help the woman and her partner to realize that these feelings are normal and that they should be expressed and not repressed.
- It is important for the woman to receive an appropriate and sympathetic explanation of what is happening at the time of the miscarriage and about what is likely to happen in the future from the doctors and nurses looking after her. For someone just to say 'better luck next time' is not appropriate.

Box 13.4 Gram-negative septicaemia

Presentation may be dramatic with pyrexia followed by hypotension and profound shock:

- Vomiting and diarrhoea may occur
- Myalgia
- Tachypnoea
- In spite of pyrexia extremities may be cyanosed and cold
- Disseminated intravascular coagulation may result
- Jaundice may develop

Investigations

- Electrolytes, urea, blood sugar, albumin, bilirubin
- Full blood count, platelets, coagulation screen, group and save serum
- Blood culture
- Cervical swab

Management

- In intensive care unit
- Appropriate blood volume replacement
- Intravenous antibiotics – a cephalosporin, gentamicin and metronidazole
- Corticosteroids may be indicated
- Appropriate treatment of complications such as coagulopathy or renal failure

Advice following a miscarriage

- To minimize the risk of infection tampons should not be used for the bleeding that occurs after a miscarriage.
- No intercourse for 2 weeks.
- Ovulation usually occurs within 3–4 weeks and so contraception should be used if necessary. Oral contraception can be started immediately.
- Probably advisable to wait 2 or 3 months before trying for another pregnancy to allow emotional and physical adjustment.

Counselling following first trimester miscarriage

- The woman's questions must be fully and sympathetically answered.
- She must be reassured that the miscarriage was not her fault and that it is normal to experience a variety of emotions for a prolonged period of time after a miscarriage.
- Following one first trimester miscarriage, the chance of the next confirmed pregnancy being successful is at least 80%; following two such miscarriages at least 70% and following three at least 50%, without any treatment. If a woman has three consecutive miscarriages investigations should be considered – see below under Recurrent miscarriages.

Second trimester miscarriage

- Much less common than first trimester miscarriage.
- A cause is more likely to be found and should be sought (Box 13.5).

Box 13.5 Some causes of second trimester miscarriage

- Structural abnormality of genital tract:
  - (1) incompetent cervix
  - (2) congenital uterine abnormality
  - (3) uterine leiomyomata (fibroids)
- Multiple pregnancy
- Fetal death in second trimester:
  - (1) chromosomal or other fetal congenital abnormality
  - (2) placental separation
  - (3) maternal infection or other illness
  - (4) rhesus disease
- Following diagnostic tests:
  - (1) amniocentesis
  - (2) fetoscopy
  - (3) cordocentesis

Incompetent cervix

- Tissues of the cervix unable to maintain closure of the internal os and miscarriage inevitably occurs, usually between 16 and 24 weeks' gestation.
- Probably responsible for approximately 10% of second trimester miscarriages.
- Usually due to instrumental dilatation of the cervix (particularly at the time of suction termination); occasionally follows dilatation of the non-pregnant cervix or cone biopsy. Rarely congenital.
- Diagnosis made from history; there are no reliable ways of diagnosing an incompetent cervix in a non-pregnant woman. Typical history is of increasing mucous discharge and a feeling of heaviness in pelvis as cervix shortens and dilates; then

with little further warning and few contractions the fetus is expelled. The fetus is the right size for dates and may be alive. The placenta may be expelled, or may be retained requiring removal under anaesthesia.

- Treatment is by insertion of Shirodkar or McDonald suture at approximately 14 weeks' gestation in the next pregnancy (by which time the likelihood of miscarriage for other reasons will have diminished).
- Occasionally possible to save the index pregnancy if the dilatation of the cervix is diagnosed in time.

Congenital uterine anomaly

- Congenital uterine anomalies occur in approximately 1% of women.
- Most women with uterine anomalies do not miscarry, but occasionally a uterine anomaly may cause recurrent miscarriages.

Uterine leiomyomata (fibroids)

Many women with fibroids become pregnant and do not miscarry, but occasionally a miscarriage may be due to a submucous fibroid or fibroid polyp.

Multiple pregnancy

There is an increased risk of pregnancy loss at all stages of gestation in a multiple pregnancy.

Causes of fetal death in second trimester

- Chromosomal or other fetal congenital abnormality.
- Placental separation (abruption).
- Maternal infection, e.g. syphilis, toxoplasmosis, rubella, cytomegalovirus (usually the fetus will not die in the second trimester with these infections but it may be born with severe congenital abnormalities).
- Other maternal illnesses, such as severe hypertension, renal disease, diabetes, lupus erythematosus, alcoholism.
- Severe rhesus incompatibility – high maternal antibody titre.

Miscarriage following diagnostic tests

- Risk of fetal loss due to amniocentesis is approximately 0.5–1%.
- Risk of fetal loss due to chorionic villus sampling is approximately 2–3%.
- Risk of fetal loss due to fetoscopy is approximately 3%.
- Risk of fetal loss due to cordocentesis is approximately 1–2%.

Management of ruptured membranes in the second trimester

For management of this condition see Box 13.6.

Box 13.6 Management of ruptured membranes in the second trimester

- Admit the woman to hospital
- Perform sterile speculum examination and take cervical swab for culture
- Perform ultrasound to determine whether the fetus is alive and if there is any abnormality
- If the fetus is dead, administer prostaglandin pessary or syntocinon infusion to encourage expulsion of the pregnancy
- If the fetus is alive advise bed rest and monitor maternal temperature and pulse rate; consider amniocentesis to allow microscopy and culture of amniotic fluid
- If there is any evidence of intrauterine infection put up a syntocinon infusion and treat with antibiotics

Special considerations in the management of second trimester miscarriages

- Try to identify cause of the miscarriage. Document sequence of events and size of fetus and whether it is macerated or not.
- If fetus appears abnormal send tissue for chromosomal analysis if fresh tissue available.
- Discuss with the woman whether she would like to see the fetus – this may be very helpful to her. Let her know what sex it is if this can be determined.
- Send fetus and placenta for pathological examination.
- Advise her to present early in the next pregnancy for appropriate surveillance and reassurance.
- Arrange follow-up appointment for discussion and counselling about 6 weeks after the miscarriage.

Recurrent miscarriages

- This term is usually used when a woman has had three or more consecutive miscarriages.
- Still unlikely that a cause for the miscarriage will be found but certain conditions should be considered (Box 13.7).

Genetic factors

- Parental chromosomal abnormalities can be found in 2–5% of couples having recurrent miscarriages. The significance of some of these abnormalities is not clear and, if an abnormality is found, the couple should be referred to a genetic counsellor.
- Other genetic factors. If a couple conceive one fetus with a neural tube defect their risk of conceiving a second fetus with a neural tube defect is 1:20.

Box 13.7 Some possible causes of recurrent miscarriages

- Genetic factors
- Cervical or uterine abnormality
- Maternal medical disorder
- Infection
- Rhesus incompatibility
- Immunological factors

- The risk of conceiving a chromosomally abnormal fetus increases with increasing age.

Cervical and uterine abnormalities, maternal medical disorders and rhesus incompatibility

These have already been discussed above under second trimester miscarriage. Cervical incompetence is the most treatable cause of second trimester miscarriage. Maternal infection is unlikely to cause recurrent miscarriages but they may rarely be associated with the presence of maternal lupus anticoagulant.

Immunological factors

There is considerable difference of opinion about the importance of immunological factors as a cause of miscarriage. The theory behind a possible immunological aetiology for recurrent miscarriage is that adequate HLA incompatibility normally allows sufficient disparity between the maternal and fetal HLA loci for maternal blocking antibodies, which prevent rejection of the foreign trophoblast to be induced. If the parents share too many HLA antigens the blocking antibody is not formed and miscarriage may occur as a result. Treatment of women with recurrent miscarriages with injections of their partner's white cells has been thought to be of benefit by some; however, there is a significant successful pregnancy rate (at least 50%) following recurrent miscarriage with no treatment and only double-blind controlled studies can give valid data.

Investigations

For investigations in a couple who have had recurrent miscarriages see Box 13.8.

Counselling of couple with recurrent miscarriages

- In most cases no cause will be identified.
- Even after three successive miscarriages the chance of the next pregnancy being successful with no treatment is well over 50%.
- Couple will require sympathetic handling and considerable reassurance before and during the next pregnancy.

Box 13.8 Possible investigations in a couple who have had recurrent miscarriages

In all cases

- Full medical, gynaecological and obstetric history
- Family history of both partners
- General and vaginal examination

In appropriate cases

- Chromosome analysis of both partners
- Hysterosalpingography or hysteroscopy
- Lupus anticoagulant screening
- Hormonal evaluation
- Blood group and antibody testing
- ? Immunological investigation

- Advise a well-balanced diet and avoidance of drugs, alcohol and smoking before and after conception.
- Bed rest and abstinence from intercourse may be helpful in early pregnancy but no definite evidence that they are.
- An early ultrasound (8 weeks) will indicate whether there is a viable pregnancy.

Ectopic pregnancy

This is a pregnancy which has implanted outside the uterine cavity, the most common sites being the ampullary or fimbrial part of the tube (75%) or the isthmus of the tube (20%) (Figure 13.3). The ratio of ectopic to continuing intrauterine pregnancies is approximately 1 to 150. The diagnosis may be very difficult to make and as the condition can be life threatening it is important to have a high index of suspicion. For the aetiology, see Box 13.9.

Box 13.9 Aetiology

- Past history of tubal infection or tubal surgery (including sterilization)
- IUCD *in situ*
- Infertility treatment such as *in vitro* fertilization and GIFT
- Idiopathic

Presentation

- Very variable depending on site of implantation; may present with tubal rupture, tubal abortion or premonitory symptoms due to tubal distension. Commonly

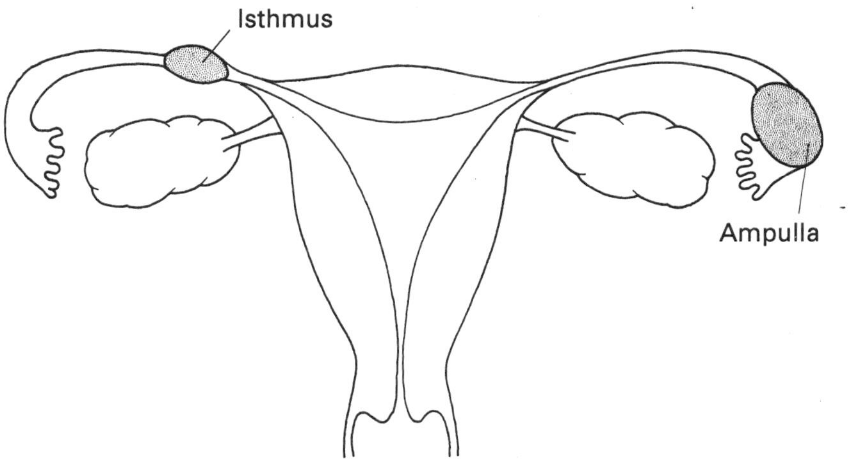

Figure 13.3 Common sites of ectopic pregnancy. (After *Miscarriage. The Facts*, G. Lachelin, 1985, Figure 4.2, Oxford University Press).

includes amenorrhoea, vaginal bleeding, lower abdominal pain and symptoms of pregnancy and may include shoulder tip pain and history of fainting.

- May present before a period has been missed.
- Laparoscopy is often indicated if ectopic is suspected and woman not shocked.
- When diagnosis very uncertain measurement of βHCG to confirm the presence of a pregnancy and ultrasound to confirm or exclude intrauterine pregnancy may be helpful. It can be very difficult to identify or to exclude an ectopic pregnancy using ultrasound. Diagnosis is easier with the new transvaginal ultrasound probes.
- Treatment is usually by salpingectomy but conservative surgery is sometimes appropriate.

Tubal rupture

- The site of implantation is usually in the narrow isthmic part of the tube.
- Tubal rupture is less common than tubal abortion, but it is very important because the woman can rapidly become shocked and may die if appropriate action is not taken.
- The woman may be unaware that she is pregnant. The duration of amenorrhoea is commonly less than 8 weeks.
- Bleeding into the peritoneal cavity causes sudden severe abdominal pain. The woman may faint and may complain of shoulder tip pain due to diaphragmatic irritation. There may be no vaginal bleeding.
- On examination the woman is shocked with pallor, low blood pressure and a thready pulse.
- The abdomen will be exquisitely tender with marked rebound tenderness.

- Do not do a vaginal examination because of risk of provoking further intraperitoneal haemorrhage.
- Insert intravenous cannula and take blood for full blood count and cross-matching. Arrange for immediate laparotomy.
- Resuscitation should take place at the same time as laparotomy as only at laparotomy can the bleeding be stopped and resuscitation without surgery will increase the haemorrhage and the likelihood of irreversible shock.
- Salpingectomy will usually be required but occasionally it may be appropriate to conserve the tube. It is important to look at the other tube to be able to give the woman some idea of the prognosis for future fertility.
- Remove as much blood as possible from the peritoneal cavity.
- Occasionally severe intraperitoneal haemorrhage will be due to persistent bleeding from the site of ovulation or to an ovarian pregnancy. The presentation will be similar and laparotomy will be required with excision of an ovarian pregnancy and repair of the ovary.
- Replace the blood that has been lost – usually between 1 and 2 litres.

Tubal abortion

- The site of implantation is usually the ampullary or fimbrial part of the tube. Bleeding into the peritoneal cavity through the fimbrial end of the tube will eventually occur.
- The woman is usually, but by no means always, aware that she is pregnant. Tubal abortion commonly presents at about 8–10 weeks' gestation.
- She will usually complain of lower abdominal pain and vaginal bleeding. She may complain of faintness and shoulder tip pain. Often, however, the symptoms will not be clear cut.
- On examination she may be pale and there may be lower abdominal tenderness. On vaginal examination there will usually be tenderness in one fornix and pain on moving the cervix.
- Salpingectomy will usually be required but occasionally it may be appropriate to conserve the tube. Check condition of the other tube.

Differential diagnosis

- Early intrauterine pregnancy with corpus luteum cyst. Ultrasound (Figure 13.4) should help to demonstrate an intrauterine pregnancy but may fail to demonstrate an extrauterine pregnancy and should not usually be used to make or exclude this diagnosis.
- Salpingitis may be associated with irregular bleeding. βHCG (human chorionic gonadotrophin) assay will show no circulating βHCG.

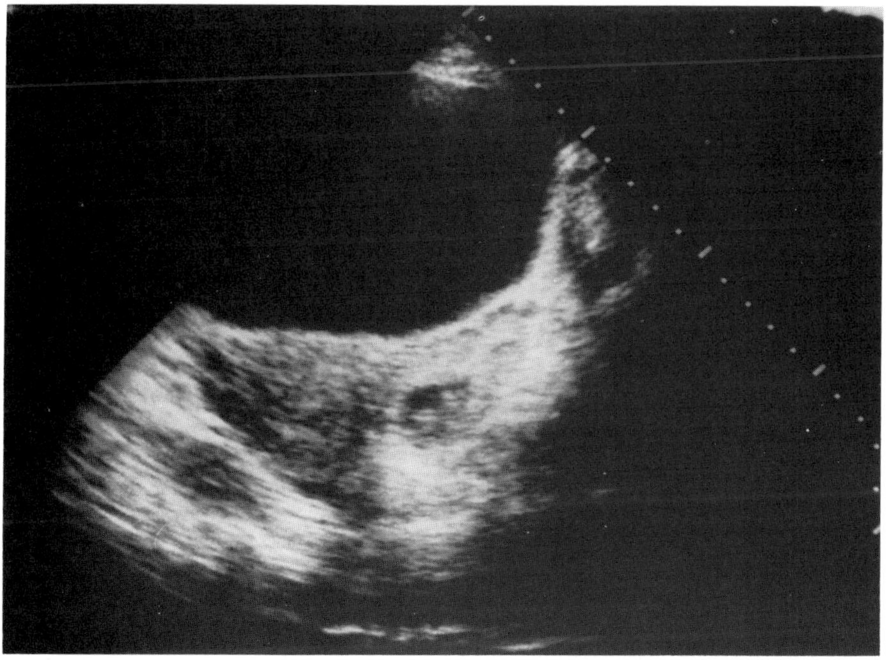

Figure 13.4 Ectopic pregnancy on ultrasound. (Courtesy of Dr Peter Twining).

- Ovulation pain. The woman will usually have experienced similar midcycle discomfort before. βHCG will be negative.
- Persistent bleeding from the site of ovulation with significant intraperitoneal haemorrhage – can be more than a litre and the presentation will then be similar to a ruptured ectopic.
- If an ectopic pregnancy is suspected, laparoscopy is usually indicated or laparotomy if the woman is shocked.

Hydatidiform mole

This is a neoplasm of the trophoblast in which there is proliferation and hydropic degeneration of the chorionic villi. For aetiology, see Box 13.10.

Presentation

- Usually presents with vaginal bleeding and sometimes passage of vesicles, although may be diagnosed on a routine ultrasound scan before bleeding has occurred.
- The uterus is usually but not always large for dates.
- Hyperemesis, severe pre-eclampsia and rarely hyperthyroidism may occur in association with a hydatidiform mole.

Box 13.10 Aetiology of hydatidiform mole

- Occurs in about 1:1500 Caucasian pregnancies but in about 1:150 pregnancies in the Far East
- Associated with chromosomal abnormality of the conceptus
- Increased incidence in older women

Complete mole – commonest type of hydatidiform mole. In more than 90% of cases the chromosomes are 46XX, with both Xs being of paternal origin; in the others the chromosomes are 46XY with both X and Y being of paternal origin. No embryo is present

Incomplete mole – the chromosomes are triploid (usually 69XXY with one maternal X and a paternal X and Y). An embryo is present initially but will often have died and disintegrated before the diagnosis is made

- The diagnosis is best made using ultrasound (Figure 13.5). With a complete mole a typical snowstorm appearance, with no amniotic sac, will be seen.
- HCG levels will usually be unduly high but they are also high in multiple pregnancy and there is an overlap between the levels in molar pregnancies and normal pregnancies.
- Bilateral theca lutein cysts commonly occur; these subside following termination of the pregnancy and fall in HCG levels.

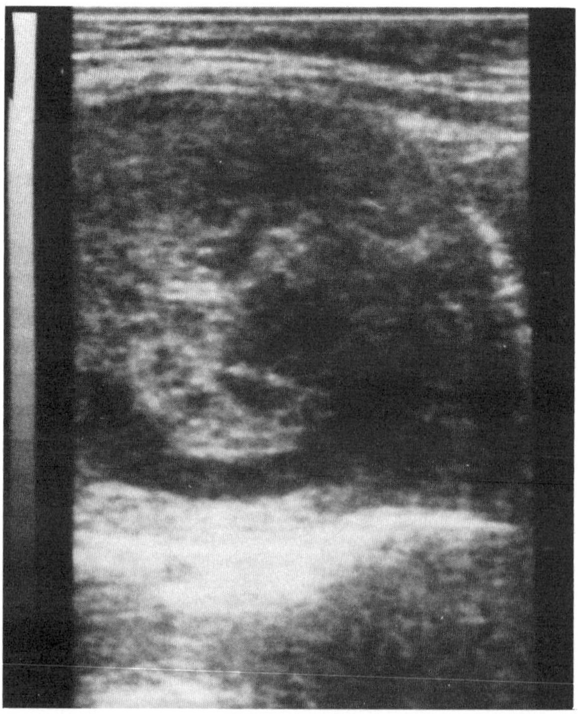

Figure 13.5 Hydatidiform mole on ultrasound. (Courtesy of Dr Peter Twining)

Management

- Once the diagnosis is made suction evacuation of the uterus should be performed. As no fetus is present with a complete mole, suction evacuation can be undertaken even when the gestation is more than 14 weeks.
- A repeat curettage 2 weeks later may be indicated.

Follow-up

- Should be organized with the appropriate supraregional centre. HCG levels are monitored fortnightly until zero (usually in less than 3 months) and then monthly, by post, for at least a year during which time pregnancy should be avoided.
- Advise barrier contraception until HCG undetectable and then oral contraception or IUCD can be used.
- Persistent molar disease occurs following approximately 10% of complete moles; it is more likely in women over 35 years old, those who are of blood group B or AB and those in whom initial HCG titre was very high.
- If HCG levels rise following evacuation of the mole or remain elevated at 3 months, refer to supraregional centre for investigation and treatment.
- The incidence of a second hydatidiform mole in a subsequent pregnancy is approximately 1:100.

Choriocarcinoma

- Occurs in about 1:20 000 pregnancies.
- Highly malignant trophoblastic tumour but can be cured by chemotherapy in the majority of cases especially if diagnosed early.
- Usually follows complete hydatidiform mole but may follow an incomplete mole, an abortion or apparently normal pregnancy or the patient may be unaware that she has conceived.
- If HCG levels remain elevated at 3 months following evacuation of a hydatidiform mole and a new pregnancy is excluded, referral to supraregional centre for consideration of chemotherapy is indicated.
- May present with continued vaginal bleeding following pregnancy or with symptoms such as cough, haemoptysis, jaundice or neurological etc. symptoms due to metastases.
- Clinical examination will include vaginal examination – the uterus may be enlarged and there may be vaginal metastases.
- Investigation will include an ultrasound scan and chest X-ray and magnetic resonance imaging if available.
- Treatment is mainly with chemotherapy, in a supraregional centre.
- Response to treatment is monitored clinically and by HCG levels.

- Pregnancy should be avoided for at least a year after successful chemotherapy.

Bleeding in early pregnancy due to problems other than pregnancy complications

Cervical ectropion

- Very common in pregnancy because of hormonal changes.
- Take cervical smear and swab for bacterial culture including *Chlamydia trachomatis*. If normal no action is indicated other than reassurance.
- If smear abnormal arrange colposcopy. Occasionally colposcopically directed biopsy will be indicated if the lesion looks suspicious. Otherwise follow-up colposcopy during pregnancy and/or 3 months post partum will be required.

Cervical polyp

- Take a smear.
- Best left untreated as removal may provoke bleeding which could be difficult to control.
- Seldom still present at postnatal check-up.

Cervical carcinoma

This may be clinically obvious or only diagnosed following smear and colposcopy. Requires urgent radical treatment.

Chapter 14
Contraception

A perfect method of contraception, applicable to all circumstances, does not exist; every known method has some disadvantages. New methods are being investigated and developed.

Box 14.1 Ideally a contraceptive method should be

- Completely safe to use with no unwanted side-effects
- 100% effective
- Easily reversible
- Simple to use, without need for medical help
- Independent of intercourse
- Inexpensive

Available methods are shown in Box 14.2; sterilization is discussed in Chapter 16. The effectiveness of different methods of contraception is expressed as the failure rate per 100 women years of exposure (Pearl index) and is calculated thus:

$$\text{Failure rate} = \frac{\text{Number of accidental pregnancies} \times 1200}{\text{Number of months of exposure}^*}$$

*10 months is deducted from the denominator for every term pregnancy and 4 months for every abortion.

The effectiveness of most methods (Box 14.2) will obviously depend on the motivation of the user. The failure rate is lower in older than in younger women as fertility decreases with age.

General approach to contraceptive counselling

- Discuss type and adequacy of contraception required, i.e. whether for family spacing or for absolute effectiveness.
- Take into consideration the age of the patient and any relevant medical condition in the patient or her partner.
- Consider the educational, cultural and religious background and personality of the patient and her partner.
- Take into consideration any local legal or other restrictions on the availability of various methods of contraception.
- A sympathetic approach with full explanation of the advantages and disadvantages of the chosen method will enhance compliance, and follow-up if required.

- Respect the informed patient's right to choose.

Box 14.2 Effectiveness of various methods of contraception

Method	*Pregnancy rate per 100 woman years*
Male sterilization	0.0–0.2
Female sterilization	0.0–0.5
Depot medroxyprogesterone acetate	0.0–1.0
Combined pill	0.1–1.0
Progestogen-only pill	0.3–5.0
IUCD	0.3–4.0
Diaphragm	2–15
Condom	2–15
Coitus interruptus	8–17
Spermicides	4–25
Fertility awareness	6–25
Contraceptive sponge	9–25
Postcoital contraception	
IUCD	Approx. 2.5
Hormonal (Yuzpe)	Approx. 25
No contraception	
Young women	80–90
Age 40	40–50
Age 45	10–20
Age 50	0–5

Fertility awareness – the 'safe' period

This method of contraception requires considerable motivation by the couple and is only effective if used conscientiously. It may, however, be the only acceptable method for a particular couple for religious or other reasons.

- The ovum can probably only be fertilized for 12–24 hours after ovulation.
- Sperms can fertilize an ovum for at least 3 days after ejaculation and possibly much longer.
- Therefore the only really 'safe' period is 2 or more days after ovulation, i.e. 3 or more days after the ovulatory rise in basal body temperature or 4 or more days after maximum ovulatory mucus secretion.

Advantages

- 'Natural' method of contraception.
- Medical help not required.
- Economical.

- Probably no adverse effects if both partners keen on the method.

Disadvantages

- Requires motivation and discipline.
- Can be difficult if cycle irregular.

Coitus interruptus (withdrawal)

Until relatively recently this was the most widely used method of contraception and most couples using this method found it acceptable.

- Only method permitted by some cultures.
- Certainly much better than no contraception and can be reasonably effective.
- Failure is usually due to failure to withdraw before ejaculation has commenced. Failure rate can be decreased by intravaginal insertion of spermicide just before intercourse.

Advantages

- Simple and always available.
- Medical help not required.
- Economical.

Disadvantages

- Many couples do not derive full satisfaction with this method and therefore find it unacceptable.

Condom

Originally used to protect against venereal disease, and in the last 200 years as a contraceptive. Still popular both in stable relationships and particularly in casual relationships. Use is increasing with awareness of AIDS.

- Additional use of spermicides increases effectiveness but not essential if couple not keen.
- Advise postcoital contraception if condom ruptures.

Advantages

- If used carefully can be very effective.
- Simple to use.
- Medical help not required.

- Some protection against gonorrhoea and trichomonal vaginitis, and probably against chlamydial infection, syphilis and AIDS. Also some protection against development of cervical neoplasia.
- Relatively inexpensive.

Disadvantages

- Motivation and discipline required. Use of condom can inhibit spontaneity and sensation.

Box 14.3 For effective use of condom

- Select reliable brand
- Apply before penetration
- Withdraw before penis becomes flaccid

Diaphragm (Figure 14.1a)

Theoretically a good method of contraception but has two main disadvantages – it is not 100% effective and its use is intercourse related. However, it is an excellent method of contraception in appropriate circumstances.

Advantages

- If used carefully, with spermicide, it is very effective.
- Can be inserted several hours before intercourse and should not interfere with satisfaction of either partner.
- Under the woman's control.
- Medical advantages include some protection against ascending infections and pelvic inflammatory disease and against development of cervical neoplasia.

Cervical and vault caps (Figure 14.1b,c,d)

These are held in place by suction, as opposed to the spring of the diaphragm, and can be useful when diaphragm unsuitable for anatomical reasons.

- Cervical cap fits over cervix.
- Vault cap covers cervix.
- Vimule used when cervix too long to allow retention of a vault cap when the use of vault cap is otherwise indicated.

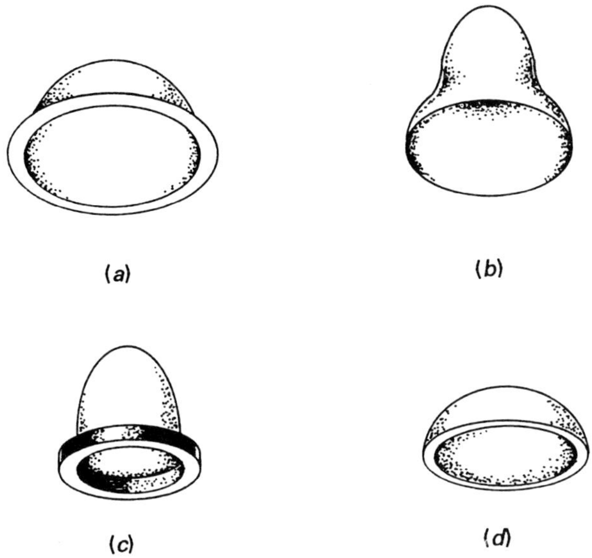

Figure 14.1 (*a*) Diaphragm; (*b*) vimule; (*c*) cervical cap; (*d*) vault cap.

Fitting of diaphragm, advice and follow-up

Fitting

- Allow time for adequate discussion and choice of method of contraception.
- Perform vaginal examination to check normality and to ensure suitability for diaphragm. If muscle tone poor or there is some degree of prolapse, a cervical or vault cap may be more suitable.
- Digitally assess the size of diaphragm required.
- Insert practice diaphragm of correct size and check the fit (Figure 14.2). Ask the woman to get up and walk about and then re-examine her.
- Help her to fit the diaphragm herself with one foot on a chair (left foot for a right-handed woman), or in squatting or lying position.
- Check position of the diaphragm and ask her to feel the correct application and to feel her cervix through the rubber – feels like the end of a nose.
- Ask her to remove the diaphragm and to re-examine the cervix no longer covered by the diaphragm.
- Show her how to apply spermicide to the diaphragm – two 1-inch (2.5 cm) strips on each side and smear some round the rim.
- Give her a practice diaphragm and spermicide to take home to practice with. Ensure she will use another method of contraception as well as the diaphragm until the next visit.

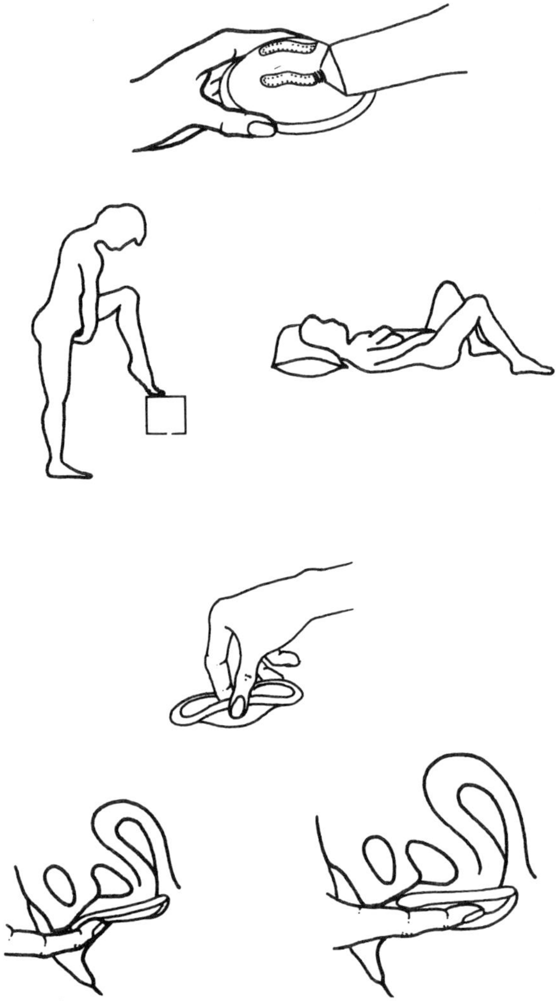

Figure 14.2 Insertion of diaphragm. (After *Contraception – Your questions answered,* J. Guillebaud, 1985, Figure 3.4, Longmans and Ortho-Cilag's *Diaphragm Patient Teaching Aid,* by permission).

- Ask her to return after a week with the diaphragm in place so that the application can be checked.

Advice

- Spermicide should always be used, and more should be inserted if intercourse takes place more than 3 hours after insertion of diaphragm or if intercourse is repeated.
- Leave the diaphragm in place for at least 6 hours after intercourse, but remove it and clean it at least once a day. After washing with soap rinse and dry it and store it in its box.
- Check the diaphragm regularly for damage.

Follow-up

- Arrange check-up with the diaphragm in place at 3 months.
- Subsequent follow-up should be every year, or sooner if any problems arise or if the woman puts on or loses more than 7 lb (3 kg) in weight, or following a pregnancy.

Female condom (Femshield)

This is a new form of barrier contraception consisting of a polyurethane sac which lines the vagina and partially covers the perineum. Acceptability and efficicacy not yet assessed. Advantages would be a combination of advantages of the diaphragm and the male condom.

Spermicides

Act by forming physical barrier to sperms and by chemical spermicidal effect.

- Various products are available in cream, foam or pessary form – important to follow instructions on timing of insertion.
- Not adequate when used on their own except in women with reduced fertility (e.g. over 45 years and/or up to 1 year postmenopausal, during lactation or in those with secondary amenorrhoea).
- Main use is in combination with another method or when 100% efficacy not essential (as in family spacing).

Box 14.4 For effective use of spermicides

- Follow instructions
- Deposit spermicide in upper third of vagina
- Allow sufficient time after insertion to become effective

Advantages

- Simple to use.
- Medical help not required.
- Under the woman's control.
- Few side-effects.

Contraceptive sponge

The idea of the contraceptive sponge is that it should occlude the cervix, soak up the sperms and kill them with spermicide contained in the sponge. However, in practice it does not effectively occlude the cervix and acts only as a spermicide.

Main use, as with spermicides, is when fertility is reduced, when 100% efficacy is not important or in combination with another method (such as coitus interruptus or IUCD).

Advantages

- Simple to use.
- Medical help not required.
- Under the woman's control.
- Active for 24 hours.
- Few side-effects.

Intrauterine contraceptive device (IUCD)

Currently used by about 4% of women in UK but rate falling because of concern about pelvic inflammatory disease. Most suitable for older woman who thinks she has completed her family. Least suitable for young nulliparous woman. The mode of action is shown in Box 14.5.

Box 14.5 Mode of action of IUCD

- Prevention of implantation
- Effectiveness enhanced by copper because of its toxic effect on sperms, blastocyst and endometrium

Advantages of IUCD

- Effective contraceptive (particularly in older women whose fertility is less than that of younger women).
- No systemic effects; serious side-effects uncommon. Most side-effects, such as menorrhagia and dysmenorrhoea, are easily treatable by removal of IUCD.
- Contraceptive effect readily reversible by removal (provided that significant infection has not occurred).
- Once inserted does not require further action by the couple for it to be effective.
- Not intercourse related, although use of spermicide should be encouraged.
- Relatively inexpensive.

Contraindications

- Abnormal bleeding from genital tract.
- Abnormality of uterine cavity – congenital or fibroids.
- Dysmenorrhoea.
- Pelvic infection or tenderness.
- Previous ectopic pregnancy or tubal surgery.
- Nulliparity.
- Valvular heart disease.
- Immunosuppression.

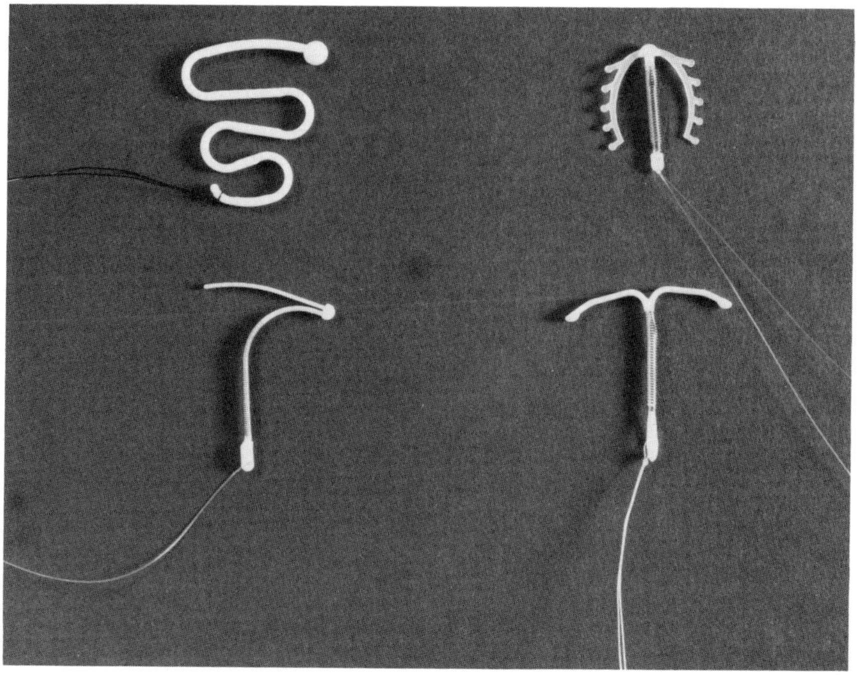

Figure 14.3 IUCDs.

Insertion of IUCD

Best inserted towards end of a period or up to day 19 of the cycle or 4–6 weeks post partum. Can be inserted at time of evacuation of uterus or termination of pregnancy, but inadvisable unless really necessary. Skilful insertion will minimize side-effects.

- Adequate counselling and discussion essential prior to insertion.
- Decide on most suitable IUCD – nowadays usually a copper device – and select correct size (Figure 14.3).

- Consider whether analgesia (mefenamic acid) or anaesthesia (paracervical block) required prior to insertion.
- Maintain verbal communication throughout insertion.
- Perform speculum and bimanual examination to check normality and to assess position of uterus.
- Re-insert speculum and hold open with screw. Clean cervix with antiseptic (Figure 14.4).

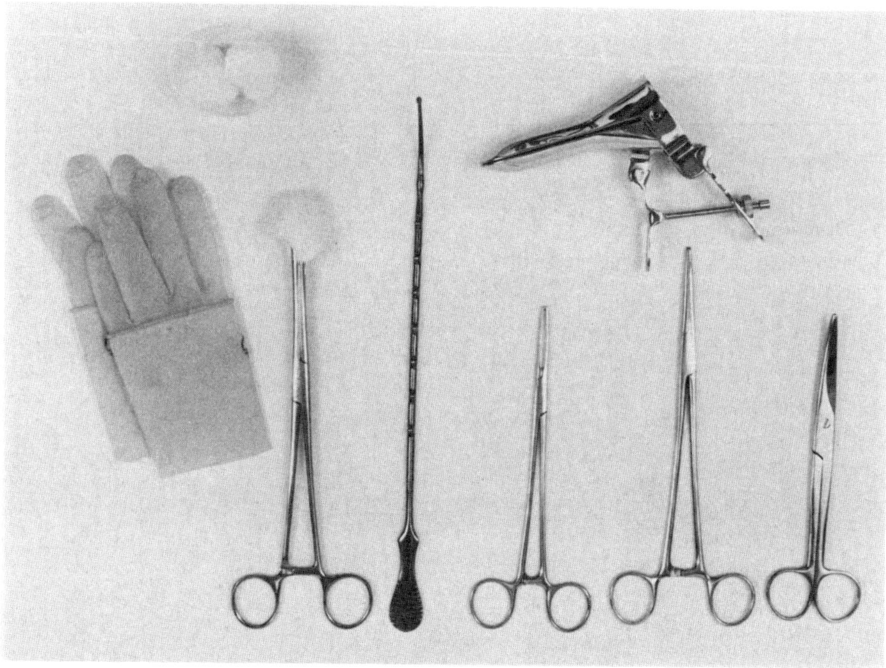

Figure 14.4 IUCD insertion set.

- Delicately pass sound to confirm direction and length of cervical canal and uterine cavity and to exclude irregularity of cavity. Application of volsellum to cervix may be necessary.
- Load device into inserter and insert according to instructions for device chosen. Take care to ensure that it is in the right plane and at the correct level in the uterus.
- Make sure the woman is able to feel the threads. She should check them after each period and use another method of contraception if unable to feel them, until she can attend for a check.
- Remind her that the method has a failure rate and of the possibility of pelvic inflammatory disease and ectopic pregnancy. Encourage her to seek medical advice if she has relevant symptoms.
- Encourage use of spermicide to decrease failure rate and incidence of infection.

- Arrange follow-up examination at 6 weeks. Check threads and palpate the end of the device with a sound and perform bimanual examination to exclude tenderness.
- Arrange annual follow-up.
- If inert can be left for as long as the woman likes if no complications.
- Copper devices are probably fully effective for at least 5 years.

Complications of IUCDs

For complications, see Box 14.6.

Box 14.6 Complications of IUCDs

- Complications at time of insertion
- Heavy or prolonged periods
- Painful periods
- Lost threads
- Expulsion
- Perforation of the uterus
- Failure – intrauterine pregnancy
- Ectopic pregnancy
- Pelvic inflammatory disease
- Subfertility

Complications at time of insertion

The drugs for use in an emergency are given in Box 14.7.

Box 14.7 Drugs for use in emergency

- Atropine 0.6 mg i.v.
- Adrenaline 1 ml 1:1000 s.c.
- Diazepam 10 mg i.v.
- Mefenamic acid 500 mg orally

Brook airway must be available

Pain

- Can be reduced by prostaglandin synthetase inhibitor (e.g. oral mefenamic acid 500 mg 1 hour before insertion) and/or paracervical block.

Vasovagal attack

- Uncommon if care taken with counselling and reassurance and if analgesia or anaesthesia are given if required.

- Causes pallor and bradycardia. Stop cervical instrumentation and remove IUCD if misplaced. Lower head of couch and give atropine 0.3 mg i.v. slowly if bradycardia persists. Give analgesia such as oral mefenamic acid 500 mg if severe discomfort persists and remove IUCD.
- Do not allow patient to go until observations are satisfactory.

Heavy or prolonged periods and painful periods

- Volume of blood lost is increased by 50–100% with an IUCD – less with smaller copper devices than with the larger plastic devices.
- Duration of bleeding is also longer with an IUCD with pre- and postmenstrual spotting.
- Pain may be due to poor fitting with an inappropriate size or to a misplaced device or to increased prostaglandin release.
- Pain and increased blood loss may be reduced by prostaglandin synthetase inhibitors such as mefenamic acid 500 mg three times daily for the first few days of the period.
- Approximately 10% of women have their IUCD removed in the first year because of bleeding and/or pain.

Lost threads

- Due to expulsion of IUCD, retraction of threads into cervical canal or uterus or perforation of uterus.
- If not pregnant attempt to 'feel' IUCD with a sound. If IUCD *in situ* advisable to remove and to replace the IUCD.
- If not pregnant and device cannot be 'felt' with a sound, advise alternative method of contraception and arrange ultrasound scan.
- If IUCD identified in uterine cavity (Figure 14.5) advise remove and replace.
- If IUCD not in uterine cavity arrange abdominal X-ray to determine whether IUCD has been expelled or uterus has been perforated.

Expulsion

- Occurs in approximately 10% of women by 1 year (50% of these within first 3 months) and is rare after 3 years. Commoner in young nulliparous than older multiparous women.
- Usually expelled during a period. Hence importance of regularly checking threads after a period.

Perforation

- Occurs in approximately 0.1% of insertions.
- Usually due to inexperience of operator. Increased risk with puerperal insertion.

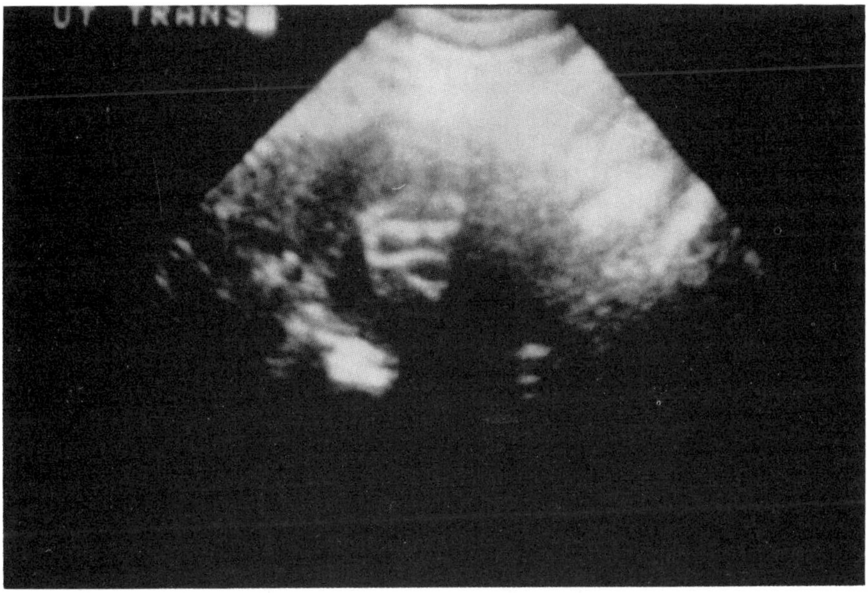

Figure 14.5 Lippes loop *in situ* on ultrasound.

- IUCD may be intraperitoneal or partially or completely in a viscus.
- Intraperitoneal plastic devices may be removable by laparoscopy, but copper-containing devices provoke adhesion formation and laparotomy is usually required.

Intrauterine pregnancy

- Increased risk of miscarriage and infection if threads visible and IUCD left *in situ*. Several maternal deaths have occurred due to infection in the second trimester.
- If threads visible and the woman wishes the pregnancy to continue, an ultrasound scan should be performed to confirm that the pregnancy is continuing normally, and the device should then be removed after counselling. A miscarriage will occasionally occur following removal of the IUCD but this will not necessarily be due to the removal.
- There is no evidence of increased risk of fetal abnormality if the device is left *in situ* but long-term outcome with copper IUCD *in situ* is not known. There may be an increased risk of pre-term rupture of the membranes and pre-term labour.

Ectopic pregnancy

- Approximately 5% of pregnancies in women with an IUCD are ectopic. Incidence increases with duration of usage and is approximately 2 per 1000 users per year.
- Increased risk is partly because IUCDs do not prevent ectopic pregnancies but do prevent a high proportion of intrauterine pregnancies, and possibly because of increased incidence of pelvic inflammatory disease with IUCDs.

- Important that IUCD users should be aware of possibility of ectopic pregnancy.
- Use of IUCD is contraindicated in a woman who has previously had an ectopic pregnancy.

Pelvic inflammatory disease

- Definite increased risk of pelvic inflammatory disease in women with IUCD. Incidence is about 2% within first year of use and increases with number of partners.
- Aseptic insertion (after treating any local infection) very important. Use of IUCD contraindicated if pelvic inflammatory disease or significant discharge present.
- Infection risk partly due to thread – multifilament worse than monofilament.
- May be associated with persistent offensive discharge.
- Infection risk is decreased if spermicide is used.
- If infection develops, cervical swab should be taken and treatment with erythromycin and metronidazole commenced. If no response to treatment within 24–48 hours IUCD should be removed, if not already taken out. Partner should be referred to department of genitourinary medicine.
- Actinomyces-like organisms are found increasingly frequently the longer an IUCD is *in situ* – in 20% of women by 5 years. If no symptoms or signs, IUCD should be removed and sent for culture and a new, usually copper, IUCD inserted.

Subfertility

- Pelvic inflammatory disease may lead to subfertility.
- One attack of pelvic inflammatory disease gives 10–15% risk of infertility due to tubal damage, two attacks increase the risk to 25–30% and three attacks to 50%.

The combined oral contraceptive (the combined pill)

The combined (oestrogen and progestogen) pill is used for contraception by more than 25% of women in the UK and by more than 50% of women under 30. Most suitable for young healthy non-smoking women who are able to remember to take the Pill regularly.

Box 14.8 Mode of action of the combined pill

- Suppression of gonadotrophin levels and therefore of follicular development and normal cyclical oestrogen and progesterone production
- Prevention of LH surge and therefore of ovulation (if a follicle does develop)
- Prevention of normal endometrial development because of suppression of cyclical oestrogen and progesterone production and because of the effect of the combined oestrogen and progestogen in the Pill
- Interference with normal cervical mucus production

Advantages of combined pill

- Very effective contraceptive.
- Reversible.
- Simple to use.
- Not intercourse related.

In addition the combined pill has several advantages other than contraceptive action:

- 'Periods' lighter and predictably regular.
- Dysmenorrhoea and premenstrual tension usually improved.
- No ovulation pain and functional ovarian cysts less common.
- Reduction in incidence of ectopic pregnancies.
- Reduction in incidence of pelvic inflammatory disease by approximately 50%.
- Possible reduction in incidence of endometriosis.
- Probable reduction in incidence of carcinoma of ovary and endometrium.

Disadvantages of combined pill

- Increased incidence of venous thromboembolism, hypertension, cerebrovascular accidents and myocardial infarction.
- Increased incidence of gallstones, cholestatic jaundice and hepatic adenoma.
- Possible increased incidence of cervical neoplasia.

Metabolic effects of the combined pill

For the metabolic effects see Box 14.9.

Contraindications to combined pill

- History of venous or arterial thrombosis, myocardial infarction or angina.
- Transient ischaemic attacks.
- Migraine.
- Significant hypertension.
- Sickle-cell disease.
- Cholestatic jaundice of pregnancy (or on the Pill).
- Abnormal liver function.
- Hepatic adenoma.
- Diabetes.
- Malabsorption syndromes.

- Serious diseases made worse by sex steroids such as breast cancer and porphyria.
- Undiagnosed bleeding from genital tract.
- Pregnancy.
- Lactation.
- Heavy smoker.
- Age more than 35 years if smokes, more than 45 if does not smoke.
- Gross obesity.
- Administration of relevant interacting drugs, e.g. enzyme inducers (see below under 'Advice for user of combined pill').

Box 14.9 Metabolic effects of combined pill

- On clotting
  - ↓ antithrombin III
  - ↑ platelet aggregation
  - ↑ fibrinolysis
  - ↑ blood viscosity
- On liver
  - ↑ blood lipids
  - ↑ transaminase
  - ↓ albumin
  - ↑ binding globulins
- On hormones
  - ↓ FSH, LH
  - ↓ endogenous oestrogen and progesterone
  - ↑ prolactin
- Factors leading to increase in blood pressure
  - ↑ angiotensin II
  - ↑ renin substrate
  - ↑ renin
  - ↑ body water
  - ↑ cardiac output

Before prescribing the combined pill

- Discuss choice of method of contraception fully.
- Exclude contraindications by careful history.
- Full general examination including breast examination and measurement of blood pressure and weight.
- Vaginal examination including cervical smear if indicated.

Choice of combined pill

The aim is to find the lowest dose pill that gives effective contraception and good cycle control with no breakthrough bleeding (BTB).

- Plasma levels of both oestrogen and progestogen in users of combined pills vary considerably from one woman to another because of differences in absorption, enterohepatic metabolism and binding; the same pill can have markedly and unpredictably different effects in different women.
- Start with a relatively low dose pill containing, e.g. 30 or 35 μg ethinyl oestradiol and a low dose of progestogen such as 500 μg norethisterone. If BTB occurs and persists give combined pill with 1000 μg norethisterone. If BTB still a problem increase the ethinyl oestradiol to 50 μg. Higher doses of progestogen are occasionally useful in women with heavy periods. (See Box 14.10.)
- Pills containing newer progestogens such as desogestrel and gestodene are currently being evaluated.

Box 14.10 Examples of pills containing increasing amounts of oestrogen and different amounts of progestogen

Pill	*Oestrogen* *Ethinyl oestradiol* (μg)	*Progestogen* *Norethisterone acetate* (μg)
Loestrin 20	20	1000
Loestrin 30	30	1500
		Norethisterone (μg)
Brevinor Ovysmen	35	500
Norinin Neocon 1/35	35	1000
Minovlar	50	1000
Gynovlar	50	3000
Anovlar	50	4000
		Levonorgestrel (μg)
Microgynon 30	30	150
Ovranette	30	150
Eugynon 30	30	250
Ovran 30	30	250
Eugynon	50	250
Ovran	50	250

Triphasic combined pills

These attempt to mimic hormonal changes of menstrual cycle more closely and to reduce the total amount of hormone taken.

Advantage

A lower total dose of hormone is required for satisfactory cycle control.

Disadvantage

They are less effective than ordinary combined pill as they are more complicated to take. Therefore less margin for error if mistakes are made.

Advice for user of combined pill

- *For immediate full effectiveness* the combined pill should be started on the first day of a period, on the day of or day after a miscarriage or abortion, 2–3 weeks post partum if not breast feeding, or on first day of 'period' or without any break if changing from progestogen-only pill or lower dose combined pill.
- *Very important not to miss a pill* particularly at end or beginning of a packet – the length of the pill-free week must not be increased as there will be a chance of follicular development if it is (Box 14.11).
- *If vomiting or diarrhoea occur* possibly resulting in failure of absorption extra precautions should be taken.
- *If treatment with an enzyme inducer* such as chlorpromazine, griseofulvin, rifampicin, spironolactone and several antiepileptics (such as barbiturates and phenytoin) is taken, this will reduce the effectiveness of the combined pill and a higher dose pill or alternative method of contraception may be necessary.
- *Symptoms that require urgent medical attention* – acute breathlessness, severe chest pain, calf pain or headache, sudden visual disturbance, difficulty in speaking, weakness or numbness of one side of the body, jaundice.
- Major surgery or treatment of varicose veins – discontinue pill but use another adequate method of contraception for 4 weeks before and 2 weeks afterwards and then recommence the pill.

Box 14.11 If a pill is missed by more than 12 hours

- Take the missed pill (or the last two missed pills if more than one was missed)
- Take the pill regularly thereafter as if no pill had been missed
- Use extra precautions for 14 days, regardless of either breakthrough or withdrawal bleeding

Follow-up

- Review at 3 months, 6 months and then annually.
- Enquire about cycle control and about possible side-effects.
- Full medical examination annually or sooner if indicated.

Progestogen-only pill (POP)

These pills contain a small amount of progestogen and have to be taken regularly at the same time every day. They are most suitable for use when oestrogen is contraindicated and fertility is somewhat reduced, e.g. by older women and those who are breast feeding. They are used by approximately 8% of women in the UK. Their mode of action is shown in Box 14.12.

Advantages of POP

- Effective if taken regularly.

- Reversible.
- Simple to use.
- Not intercourse related.
- Few side-effects other than on bleeding pattern.
- Can be used by those for whom oestrogen is contraindicated.
- Probable reduction in incidence of pelvic inflammatory disease.

Disadvantages of POP

- *Must* be taken regularly at the same time each day.
- Cycle irregularity and/or breakthrough bleeding occurs in many women.
- Possible increase in incidence of ectopic pregnancies.

Box 14.12 Mode of action of POP

- Alteration of quality of cervical mucus, making it resistant to sperm penetration
- Prevention of normal endometrial development
- Interference with ovulation in many cycles

Metabolic effects of POP

- Not as well studied as those of combined pill but appears to have few metabolic effects.
- Apparently no effect on clotting mechanisms.
- Probably minimal if any effect on lipids.
- Probably minimal if any effect on carbohydrate metabolism – therefore suitable for use by diabetics.
- No effect on blood pressure.

Indications for use of POP as opposed to combined pill

- Older women – non-smokers over 45 years old and smokers over 35.
- During lactation.
- Many diabetics (but not those at highest risk for arterial disease).
- Obese women.
- Sickle-cell disease.
- Women with hypertension.
- Some other women with contraindications to oestrogen use, such as those with history of venous thrombosis and some of those with migraine.

Contraindications to use of POP

- History of arterial thrombosis or high risk of arterial disease.
- Hepatic adenoma.
- Severe liver disease.
- Malabsorption syndromes.
- Possibly some sex steroid dependent cancers.
- Unreliable pill taker.
- Undiagnosed genital tract bleeding.
- Pregnancy.
- Previous ectopic pregnancy.
- History of recurrent functional ovarian cysts.
- Administration of relevant interacting drugs, e.g. enzyme inducers (see above).

Before prescribing POP

- Discuss choice of method of contraception fully.
- Exclude contraindications.
- Ensure that woman aware of need to take POP absolutely regularly at same time each day.
- Full general examination including breast examination and measurement of blood pressure and weight.
- Vaginal examination including cervical smear if indicated.
- Discuss possible side-effects.

Box 14.13 Choice of POP

Progestogen	μg
Norethisterone	350
Ethynodiol acetate	500
Levonorgestrel	30

No clear benefit of prescribing one rather than another; ethynodiol acetate is the most progestogenic of the three

Advice for user of POP

- It is *essential* that the pills are taken regularly every 24 hours – best taken in the morning if intercourse normally takes place in the evening as effect on mucus is beginning to wear off at 24 hours.
- If menstruating start on first day of period and use extra precautions such as sheath for first 7 days as may take a week to be fully effective.

- Post partum can be started any time in first 2–3 weeks without the need for extra precautions. If lactating start after a week to allow lactation to become established.
- If started on day of or day following miscarriage or abortion there is no need for extra precautions.
- If changing from combined pill start immediately after a course and then no need for extra precautions.
- If taking of a pill delayed by 3 hours or more another method of contraception should be used as well for 2 days.
- If vomiting or diarrhoea occur possibly resulting in failure of absorption, extra precautions should be taken.

Follow-up

- Review at 3 months, 6 months and then annually.
- Enquire about cycle control and possible side-effects.
- Full medical examination annually or sooner if indicated.

Depot medroxyprogesterone acetate – DMPA (Depot-Provera)

This is given by deep intramuscular injection – 150 mg – every 12 weeks. Very effective contraceptive particularly suitable for those who find it difficult to take pills regularly. Used by less than 1% of women in the UK, but by several million world wide. Its mode of action is given in Box 14.14.

Box 14.14 Mode of action of DMPA

- Prevention of ovulation
- Prevention of normal endometrial development
- Alteration of cervical mucus making it resistant to sperm penetration

Advantages of DMPA

- Very effective.
- Few metabolic effects; no serious side-effects.
- Reversible.
- Simple to administer and once given does not require any further action for it to be effective.
- Not intercourse related.
- Inexpensive.

In addition DMPA has several advantages other than contraceptive action:

- 'Periods' lighter and may stop altogether.

- Dysmenorrhoea and premenstrual tension usually improved.
- No ovulation pain.
- Reduction in incidence of ectopic pregnancies.
- Reduction in incidence of pelvic inflammatory disease.
- Probable reduction in incidence of endometriosis.

Disadvantages of DMPA

- Irreversible for 2–3 months and return of ovulatory cycles and fertility may be delayed for at least a year.
- Irregular bleeding in some women.
- Weight gain of several pounds commonly occurs.
- Masculinization of female fetus if given in pregnancy.

Indications for DMPA

- Women seeking hormonal method of contraception in whom oestrogen is contraindicated and/or who would not take pills regularly.
- Sickle-cell disease.
- Short-term contraception, e.g. before and after vasectomy until azoospermia confirmed and at time of post partum rubella vaccination.

Contraindications to DMPA

- History of arterial thrombosis or high risk of arterial disease.
- Migraine.
- Hepatic adenoma or severe liver disease.
- Possibly some sex steroid dependent cancers.
- Undiagnosed genital tract bleeding.
- Pregnancy.

Before prescribing DMPA

- Discuss choice of method of contraception fully.
- Exclude contraindications.
- Full general examination including breast examination and measurement of blood pressure and weight.
- Vaginal examination including cervical smear if indicated.
- Discuss possible side-effects particularly irregular bleeding, amenorrhoea, weight gain and delay in return of fertility (9 months on average).

Mode of administration

- Give before day 5 of menstrual cycle if menstruating or within 5 days of first trimester miscarriage or abortion.
- Give more than 5 weeks post partum or post second trimester abortion so as to minimize side-effects of bleeding.
- Give by deep intramuscular injection into upper outer quadrant of buttock and do not massage the injection site as massage reduces the duration of effectiveness.
- Repeat injection every 3 months if required.

Follow-up

- Review at 3 months or sooner if necessary.
- Full medical examination annually or sooner if indicated.

Postcoital contraception

The aim of postcoital contraception is to prevent implantation if fertilization occurs. Implantation normally takes place 5–7 days after conception (but probably fails to occur for at least 30% of fertilized ova under normal circumstances). The methods are given in Box 14.15.

Box 14.15 Methods of postcoital contraception

- Ethinyl oestradiol 100 μg + levonorgestrel 500 μg within 72 hours of first episode of unprotected intercourse in current cycle; repeated 12 hours later (Yuzpe regimen)
- Insertion of IUCD within 5 days of unprotected intercourse (or within 5 days of ovulation if several episodes of unprotected intercourse in current cycle)
- *Essential* that woman is seen again at or before 3 weeks after treatment

Effectiveness

Success rate for Yuzpe regimen varies with time in cycle of exposure – approximately 1–4% of women become pregnant. With IUCD method only about 1 in 500 women become pregnant.

Complications of treatment

- Nausea and vomiting may occur with Yuzpe regimen and lead to failure.
- Risks of IUCD are those of IUCD insertion.
- Possibility of ectopic pregnancy may be increased with postcoital contraception.
- Continuing pregnancy, particularly if inaccurate history obtained.

Contraindications to postcoital contraception

- Pregnancy.
- Contraindications to Yuzpe regimen include any absolute contraindication to oestrogen therapy.
- Contraindications to IUCD include several of those discussed under IUCD as a method of contraception (see above).

Procedure

- Accurate history of date of last period and of all days of unprotected intercourse in current cycle essential. Normal cycle length and current method of contraception important. Exclude any contraindications to either method of postcoital contraception. Discuss and decide on future method of contraception.
- Perform vaginal examination.
- If no contraindication and if not already too late, discuss and decide on method of postcoital contraception.
- Make sure the woman understands the vital necessity of returning in 3 weeks, or sooner if any problems such as vomiting, pain or persistent or heavy bleeding occur.

Chapter 15

Therapeutic abortion

Since the Abortion Act of 1967, termination of pregnancy in the United Kingdom is legal if two registered medical practitioners are of the opinion formed in good faith that:

1. The continuance of the pregnancy would involve risk to the life of the pregnant woman greater than if the pregnancy were terminated.
2. The continuance of the pregnancy would involve risk of injury to the physical or mental health of the pregnant woman greater than if the pregnancy were terminated.
3. The continuance of the pregnancy would involve risk of injury to the physical or mental health of the existing child(ren) of the family of the pregnant woman greater than if the pregnancy were terminated.
4. There is a substantial risk that if the child were born it would suffer from such physical or mental abnormalities as to be seriously handicapped.

- A 'green form' (Certificate A) must be completed and signed by the two registered medical practitioners who agree that the termination should be performed.
- A 'white' form must be completed and signed by the medical practitioner (who need not be one of those signing the green form) who performs the termination of pregnancy.
- The woman's signed informed consent is mandatory, but the partner's consent is not necessary although it is obviously preferable, if they are in a stable relationship.
- The above clauses are not accepted by everyone. Therapeutic abortion is a controversial issue and religious, cultural and individual sensitivities of patients, medical practitioners and nurses must be respected.
- In other countries laws on abortion range from absolute prohibition to abortion on demand.
- In this country more than 100 000 terminations are carried out each year, the majority under Clause 2.
- The gestation limit for abortion is currently under review in the United Kingdom. It has been suggested by some that it should be 24 weeks for congenital abnormalities but lower for other indications.

History and counselling

- A sympathetic and supportive approach is required. Practitioners who do not accept the concept of therapeutic abortion should be able to refer the patient to a colleague who does not hold similar views.
- An adequate history (including a full medical, obstetric and gynaecological history)

must be obtained and an attempt must be made to establish the reason for the occurrence of the unwanted pregnancy (e.g. failed contraception, ignorance or a failed relationship) in order that suitable advice can be given about preventing an unwanted pregnancy in the future.

- Inconvenience is not an indication for termination of pregnancy and it is usually more appropriate for the woman to continue the pregnancy if she is in a stable relationship in which she intends to have children, albeit at a slightly later date. Much unhappiness is caused when termination done in these circumstances is followed by failure to conceive at a later date.
- It is important to establish that the patient is not seeking termination because of a misconception, e.g. that it would be medically dangerous for her to remain pregnant or that she is unlikely to be able to have a healthy baby having had an obstetric problem in the past.
- Alternatives to abortion must be fully explored and the patient must be given adequate time to consider these.
- If the patient is under age, a parent or guardian must be involved in the discussion and must give his or her signed consent if the termination is decided upon.
- If termination is being considered on medical grounds or because of suspected fetal abnormality, the patient must be fully counselled as to the risks of continuing the pregnancy or the likely problems that would be encountered by the baby if the pregnancy were to continue. A woman undergoing termination of pregnancy for medical or fetal reasons will need even more support than one undergoing termination of an unwanted normal pregnancy.
- The patient must be made aware of what the procedure entails and of the possible risks of the procedure.
- It is usually appropriate to warn her that cervical damage and uterine perforation or rupture (necessitating laparotomy) occasionally occur and that readmission for evacuation of retained products of conception is sometimes required.
- It is important that future contraception should be fully discussed.
- It is not usually appropriate to perform sterilization at the time of therapeutic abortion as there is a greater chance that the woman will regret the decision. There is also a higher failure rate.
- If the medical practitioner considers that termination of pregnancy is not indicated the reasons must be stated to the patient and arrangements for care and support during pregnancy must be offered.

Examination

- A general and vaginal examination must be performed and the length of gestation established.
- A cervical smear should be taken if indicated.
- A cervical swab should be taken for detection of chlamydial infection and for other organisms if there is evidence of or a particular likelihood of infection.

Other investigations

- Blood should be taken for haemoglobin estimation and for blood grouping to determine whether the woman is rhesus positive or negative and for other tests as appropriate.
- An ultrasound scan may be indicated if it is not possible to establish the gestation by examination or if the uterus is large for dates. The patient should usually be protected from seeing the scan if a decision to terminate the pregnancy has already been made.

Methods of termination of pregnancy

- *First trimester termination* is usually achieved by suction termination (Figure 15.1) but medical termination of pregnancy using an antiprogesterone (RU486) followed 48 hours later by a prostaglandin pessary is currently being evaluated.

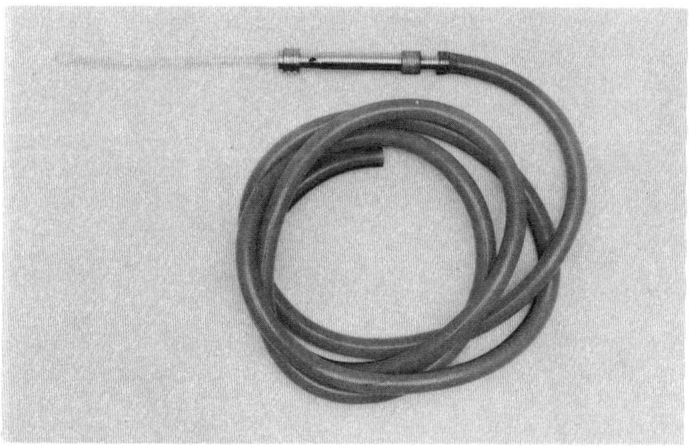

Figure 15.1 Karmen cannula for suction termination.

- *Second trimester termination* can be achieved by intra- or extra-amniotic instillation of prostaglandin, by dilatation and evacuation or by hysterotomy.

First trimester suction termination

- Suction termination is preferable to dilatation and curettage as the complication rate is much lower.
- Can be performed using local anaesthesia (paracervical block) or general anaesthesia.
- The insertion of a prostaglandin pessary 3–4 hours before surgery will soften the cervix and reduce the likelihood of cervical trauma.
- Following appropriate anaesthesia the cervix is dilated to accommodate a suction cannula of appropriate diameter. The diameter (in mm) required corresponds approximately to the gestation in weeks. Dilatation beyond 10 mm should be

avoided especially in nulliparous patients as cervical damage is likely to occur with greater dilatation.

Complications include anaesthetic complications, uterine perforation, cervical damage, incomplete abortion, haemorrhage and infection. These complications should occur infrequently. Long-term complications include regret and depression, infertility, midtrimester miscarriage and rhesus isoimmunization.

Second trimester abortion

- This is currently usually achieved using intra- or extra-amniotic prostaglandin, with adequate analgesia such as an epidural anaesthetic; dilatation and evacuation, usually under general anaesthesia; or occasionally hysterotomy under general anaesthesia.
- *Intra-amniotic prostaglandin termination* is performed under ultrasound control, usually with an epidural block for analgesia. Amniocentesis is performed and approximately 200 ml amniotic fluid is removed prior to the instillation of prostaglandin and urea (given to ensure that the fetus is not alive when it is aborted – unless fetal tissue is required to make or confirm a diagnosis in a case of fetal abnormality). If the uterus fails to contract by 12 hours, a second dose of prostaglandin can be administered or a syntocinon infusion (20 units in 500 ml Hartmann's solution) can be commenced. A strict fluid balance chart must be kept because the antidiuretic action of syntocinon can lead to water intoxication. Exploration of the uterus should usually be performed following abortion unless the products have been completely aborted. It can be done under epidural anaesthesia.
- *Extra-amniotic prostaglandin termination* involves the instillation of prostaglandin via a Foley catheter inserted through the cervical canal into the extra-amniotic space. Syntocinon infusion is seldom required but may be given to expedite abortion. Exploration of the uterus should usually be performed following abortion.
- *Dilatation and evacuation* is usually performed under general anaesthesia with ultrasound control to ensure that the uterus is empty at the end of the procedure. The cervix should be softened preoperatively with prostaglandin or hydrophilic laminaria. Cervical damage is likely if this procedure is performed by an unskilled operator.
- *Hysterotomy* is seldom performed nowadays as it carries a higher morbidity including a greater risk of pulmonary embolism than the other procedures.

Complications of second trimester termination include anaesthetic complications, intravasation of prostaglandins, uterine rupture, cervical damage, incomplete abortion, haemorrhage and infection. Long-term complications include regret and depression, infertility and rhesus isoimmunization. The mortality rate of second trimester abortion is higher than that of first trimester abortion.

Assessment before allowing patient home

- Suction termination and dilatation and evacuation are often performed on a day case basis.

- Ensure patient has recovered from whatever anaesthetic she was given.
- Check that abdomen is soft and not tender and that vaginal bleeding is not heavy.
- Ensure that anti-D immunoglobulin (250 units) is given if patient is rhesus negative.
- Make sure that she has had appropriate contraceptive advice. The combined contraceptive pill can be started straightaway to ensure full protection in the following cycle. Intercourse should not be resumed until after a period or withdrawal bleed has occurred.
- Provide an opportunity for further counselling if required.

Complications following therapeutic abortion

Women requesting termination of pregnancy should be aware that complications such as the following can occur:

- Anaesthetic complications (uncommon).
- Perforation or rupture of the uterus (uncommon). Laparotomy is required.
- Bleeding which sometimes requires re-evacuation of the uterus (approximately 2%).
- Infection – often related to preceding infection (approximately 2%).
- Regret, depression and psychosexual problems (not uncommon).
- Subfertility.
- Cervical incompetence with midtrimester miscarriage in next pregnancy.
- Rhesus isoimmunization (much less common now anti-D immunoglobulin available).

Chapter 16
Sterilization

- Voluntary sterilization is a popular method of birth control in many parts of the world.
- When chosen appropriately it is a very satisfactory method of contraception.
- It allows freedom from having to use other methods of contraception and from their side-effects.
- It should, however, only be chosen after careful consideration and when permanent contraception is required.
- There is a small failure rate and the woman must be aware of this.
- Sterilization is not condoned by certain religious groups such as Roman Catholics and Orthodox Jews.

Important points in history from a woman requesting sterilization

- *Reasons for request* – usually because she feels she does not want more, or sometimes any, children but may be because of medical or psychiatric illness or for eugenic reasons.
- *Previous methods of contraception* and reasons why other methods of contraception are not acceptable. She may not have fully considered alternative methods.
- *Age of patient* – if under 30 years old need to be extra certain that she is making the right choice, if over 40 years old alternative methods of contraception may be adequate and more appropriate.
- *Previous obstetric history* – important to make sure she is making the choice because she does not want more children and not because she has a mistaken idea that there is a contraindication to her having further pregnancies or that further pregnancies are unlikely to be successful. A nulliparous woman will occasionally request sterilization: it is very important to be sure that she is making the right choice.
- *Marital status* – it is important to find out if the woman is in a stable relationship to try to reduce the likelihood that she will regret being sterilized. The husband/partner's consent is not required by law, but it is wise to ensure that he is in favour of sterilization to reduce the likelihood of subsequent disharmony.
- *Menstrual history* including that prior to taking the contraceptive pill if she is currently taking the Pill. It would not, for example, be appropriate to sterilize a woman with menorrhagia who has completed her family.
- *Full gynaecological history* – previous surgery or pelvic sepsis, fibroids or prolapse may influence the management.

- *Psychosexual and social history* is very important. Sterilization is unlikely to resolve psychosexual problems or to save a marriage.

Examination

General and vaginal examination must be performed to exclude any contraindication to sterilization and to decide the best approach (e.g. laparoscopy, minilaparotomy or occasionally vaginal route).

Counselling

- Request for sterilization must be the woman's own choice without coercion of any kind.
- All alternatives must be thoroughly considered, including vasectomy.
- If she chooses to be sterilized she should do so thinking of the procedure as a permanent irreversible method of contraception. She must consider the, albeit remote, possibility of marital breakdown or death of her partner or children.
- The procedure should be carefully explained and any queries answered as many people are unaware what sterilization means. It should be emphasized that it is a mechanical block to the passage of the egg (which is very small and will be absorbed) along the tube and that it will not of itself alter ovarian, menstrual or sexual function, other than by causing infertility.
- If she is currently taking the combined contraceptive pill she must be warned that her periods are likely to become heavier when she stops taking it; if she currently has an IUCD her periods may become lighter when it is removed.
- She must be aware that there is a failure rate of approximately 0.5% and that an ectopic pregnancy can occur.
- Particularly careful counselling must be given to a pregnant woman who requests sterilization. The failure and request for reversal rate are higher when sterilization is performed at the time of caesarean section or following termination of pregnancy. If a request is made at the beginning of a pregnancy in which an elective caesarean section is planned and careful counselling is given, it may be reasonable to perform sterilization at the time of caesarean section if the baby seems to be healthy but the woman must be aware that it is impossible to be certain that a baby is completely healthy at birth, and that it will survive infancy. Sterilization at the time of unexpected caesarean section or termination of pregnancy is inadvisable and it is usually better to wait 2 or 3 months.
- Very careful counselling must be given to a nulliparous woman requesting sterilization.

Sterilization techniques

- Can be performed by laparoscopy, minilaparotomy or by vaginal route.

- Can be performed on day case or inpatient basis.
- The lumen of the fallopian tubes may be interrupted by the application of clips or rings, by diathermy or by excision of part or all of the tube. Clips cause the least damage to the tube and allow the best chance of reversal. Diathermy causes considerable damage and complete excision precludes the possibility of reversal.

Laparoscopic sterilization

- Can be done as a day case.
- General, local or regional anaesthesia.
- Bladder must be empty.
- Verres needle introduced carefully to create pneumoperitoneum with carbon dioxide or nitrous oxide.
- Trocar and cannula then introduced, usually subumbilically.
- Laparoscope introduced via cannula and pelvis inspected.
- Second trocar and cannula introduced.
- Clip applicator or diathermy forceps introduced via cannula.

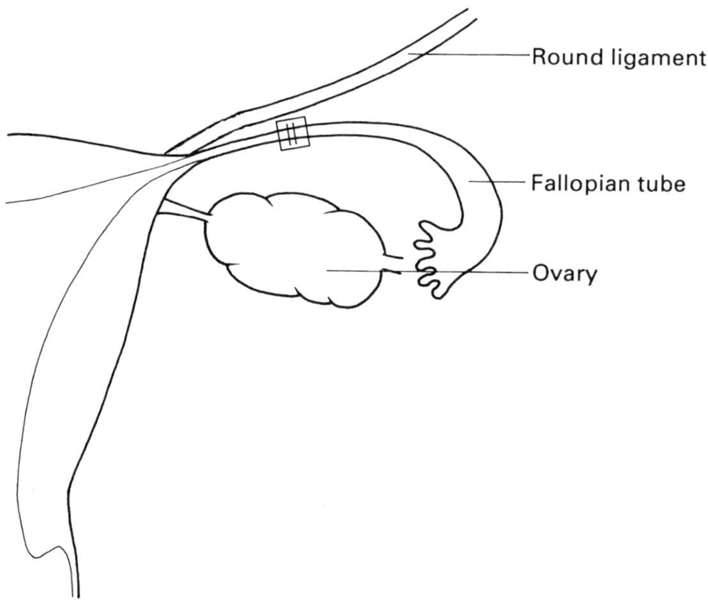

Figure 16.1 Clip on fallopian tube.

- Tubes very carefully identified by visualizing cornual and fimbrial ends and then clipped (or diathermied) approximately 1.5 cm from cornua of uterus (Figure 16.1).
- Procedure checked.

- Gas expelled.
- Incision closed with subcuticular absorbable suture.

Minilaparotomy

- Advantage is that it can be performed by those not trained to perform laparoscopy. It is a simpler, cheaper and safer procedure in the less developed countries, where paramedics are taught to perform sterilization.
- Can be performed with general, regional or local anaesthesia.
- Bladder must be empty.
- Uterus can usefully be elevated with a pack in the vagina.
- Small suprapubic incision.
- Fallopian tubes identified and clipped, or ligated and piece excised (Pomeroy sterilization).
- Wound closed with subcuticular absorbable suture material.

Box 16.1 Before a woman is sent home following a laparoscopic or minilaparotomy sterilization

- Ensure she is fully recovered from the anaesthetic
- Exclude intra-abdominal tenderness
- If she has shoulder tip pain explain that this is due to gas under the diaphragm
- Advise her to report back if any problems are experienced
- Remind her of the failure rate and possibility of an ectopic pregnancy and advise her to seek medical advice early if she misses a period

Immediate complications of sterilization

- Can be due to anaesthesia or to surgery and are more likely to occur with less skilled operator and with laparoscopy than with minilaparotomy.
- As laparoscopy is an initially blind procedure all intrabdominal structures are at risk of damage unless adequate precautions are taken. Imperative that any damage is recognized and appropriate action is taken.

Long-term sequelae

- Failure rate of approximately 0.5% – the pregnancy may be intrauterine (usually) or ectopic.
- Loss of chance of pregnancy may cause loss of libido.

- Some women will regret sterilization and some will ask for reversal, usually because of changed circumstances.

Reversal of sterilization

- Determine the reason for the request.
- Adequate counselling is very important.
- Discuss implications of reversal of sterilization including the small risk associated with a laparotomy, the likelihood of successful reversal, the risk of an ectopic pregnancy and the possible complications that could arise with an intrauterine pregnancy.
- The likelihood of successful reversal will depend on the type of sterilization procedure that was performed and information about this must be obtained. With a clip sterilization and normal tubes in a young woman the success rate is over 80%; with diathermy sterilization successful reversal is unlikely.
- There is an increased risk of ectopic pregnancy following reversal of sterilization.
- The possible complications of an intrauterine pregnancy depend on many factors but the age of the patient and her medical and obstetric history are clearly important. If she is approaching 40 years of age she must be warned of her decreased chance of conception, and increased likelihood of miscarriage, and the increased risk of a chromosomally abnormal fetus.
- A full general and a vaginal examination must be performed to exclude any contraindications to surgery or to pregnancy.
- If reversal of sterilization is contemplated evidence of ovulation (basal body temperature chart) and normal spermatogenesis (semen analysis) must be obtained. The woman's rubella status must be ascertained.
- If reversal is not technically feasible and pregnancy is not contraindicated, the possibility of *in vitro* fertilization should be discussed.

Vasectomy

- Vasectomy is a popular form of permanent contraception in many countries.
- The technique is simple and serious complications are uncommon; vasectomy is therefore particularly suited to less developed countries.

Counselling

- Request for sterilization must be the man's own choice with no coercion of any kind.
- All alternatives must be thoroughly considered.
- If he chooses to be sterilized he should do so thinking of the procedure as a

permanent irreversible method of contraception. He must consider the, albeit remote, possibility of marital breakdown or death of his partner or children.

- Particular care must be taken in counselling young or unattached men.
- The marital status is important. His partner's consent is not required by law but it is wise to ensure that she is in favour of sterilization to reduce the likelihood of subsequent marital disharmony.
- The procedure should be carefully explained and any queries answered as many people are unaware what vasectomy means. It should be explained that it is a mechanical block to the passage of the sperms which are very small and will be absorbed and that it will not of itself alter sexual function other than by causing infertility.
- It is important that the possible psychosexual effects of vasectomy should be considered.
- The couple must be aware that there is a failure rate (less than 1%) and that recanalization can occur.

Procedure

- Usually performed on an outpatient basis under local anaesthesia.
- Variety of techniques which involve division and usually resection of a portion of the vasa deferentia.
- Some postoperative discomfort is normal and the patient should be advised to rest for 24 hours after surgery and to avoid strenuous exercise for a week and to abstain from intercourse for two weeks.
- Semen analysis should be performed after about 20 ejaculations. Before the vasectomy can be deemed successful two semen analyses performed about a week apart must be azoospermic.

Complications

- Haematoma formation is not uncommon. Usually resolves without drainage.
- Infection is less common.
- Sperm granuloma may form. Usually resolves spontaneously but occasionally may require excision.
- Psychosexual problems such as impotence may ensue.
- Antisperm antibodies commonly occur and reduce successful pregnancy rate after vasectomy reversal, even when patency is obtained, to less than 50%.

Chapter 17
Non-malignant conditions of the vulva, vagina and cervix

Vulva

Box 17.1 Non-malignant conditions of the vulva

Benign cysts and tumours

- Associated with Bartholin's gland – cyst, abscess and adenoma
- Sebaceous cysts
- Cyst of canal of Nuck
- Lipoma
- Papilloma
- Fibroma
- Pigmented naevus
- Neurofibroma
- Hidradenoma
- Urethral caruncle

Vulval dystrophies

- Vulval atrophy
- Hypoplastic dystrophy (lichen sclerosus)
- Hypertrophic dystrophy and leukoplakia
- Mixed dystrophy

Behçet's syndrome

Vulval varicosities

Vulval infections and warts (see Chapter 7)

Benign cysts and tumours

Cyst and abscess associated with Bartholin's gland

- Arise from blockage and dilatation of duct of Bartholin's gland.
- Lie posterolateral to vaginal introitus and may bulge into introitus.
- If uninfected may be asymptomatic.

- When infected an acutely painful Bartholin's abscess may form.
- Treatment is by marsupialization.

Adenoma of Bartholin's gland

- Rare and may be macroscopically indistinguishable from malignant adenocarcinoma.
- Excision and histological examination required.

Sebaceous cysts

- Arise from blockage of ducts of sebaceous glands usually between labia majora and minora. Contain cheesy material. Usually resolve spontaneously but occasionally require surgical incision or excision.

Cyst of canal of Nuck

- Part of processus vaginalis may persist beneath anterior part of labium majus or in the groin and a cyst may form. Rare.

Lipoma, papilloma, fibroma, pigmented naevus, neurofibroma

- Any of these and other benign tumours may arise in the vulva.
- Treatment is surgical with histological examination if they cause symptoms or there is doubt about their nature.

Hidradenoma

- Sweat gland tumour.
- Typically forms pea-sized raised nodule with red top.
- Treatment is by excision and histological examination.

Urethral caruncle

- Bright red painful polypoidal pea-sized lesion arising from posterior margin of urethral meatus.
- Causes acute discomfort and dysuria and occasionally bleeds.
- Must be differentiated from prolapsed urethral mucosa and urethral diverticulum which should be managed by a urologist.
- Treatment is by biopsy and cautery or diathermy.

Vulval dystrophies

Vulval atrophy

- Usually occurs after the menopause but may occur earlier.

- Vulval skin becomes thin and shiny and introitus is stenosed.
- Histologically the epidermis is thin and there is hyalinization of the dermis.
- Occasionally treatment with oestrogen may be beneficial but often it is not.
- Patient should be followed up as hypertrophic changes may occur and biopsy should then be performed.

Hypoplastic dystrophy (lichen sclerosus)

- Usually postmenopausal but occasionally occurs in children and young adults.
- Areas of white or pink skin which ultimately become atrophic with a waxen appearance.
- Histologically there is hyperkeratosis and the rete pegs are flat.
- Often presents with pruritus.
- Biopsy usually necessary to make the diagnosis and to exclude premalignant or malignant change.
- Pruritus may be relieved by corticosteroid cream and systemic antihistamines.
- Patient must be followed up because malignant change may occur.

Hypertrophic dystrophy and leukoplakia

- Patches of white hypertrophied skin are present.
- Histologically, there is hyperkeratosis and the rete pegs of the epidermis dip deeply into the dermis.
- Pruritus may be relieved as above.
- Biopsy is mandatory and careful follow-up is essential.
- Local excision occasionally required.

Other vulval dystrophies

- Other premalignant and malignant conditions of the vulva such as vulval intraepithelial neoplasia, Bowen's disease, Paget's disease and frank carcinoma may occur. Biopsy of any suspicious lesion is mandatory.

Behçets syndrome

- Uncommon condition in which painful shallow ulcers occur on the vulva and in the mouth. Other systemic manifestations may occur.
- Aetiology unknown.
- Ulcers heal spontaneously but then recur. No known effective treatment.

Vulval varicosities

- These are seldom symptomatic except during pregnancy when they should be controlled by supportive measures.
- If they are symptomatic outside pregnancy surgical referral may be appropriate.

Pruritus vulvae

Intense itching of the vulva may be due to one of the conditions specified in Box 17.2.

Box 17.2 Pruritus vulvae

Infections

- *Candida albicans*
- *Trichomonas vaginalis*
- Tinea cruris
- Pediculosis pubis
- Threadworms

Local dermatological conditions

- Vulval dystrophies
- Premalignant and malignant conditions of the vulva

Local reaction to chemical substances

- Glycosuria
- Caps, condoms, contraceptive creams
- Soap, soap powder, bath salts, deodorants
- Medications used to treat pruritus

General dermatological conditions

- Allergic dermatitis
- Psoriasis
- Scabies

General medical conditions

- Diabetes
- Drug allergy
- Jaundice
- Uraemia
- Leukaemia

Psychosomatic conditions

Treatment of pruritus vulvae if above causes excluded

- Loose cotton underwear
- Local hydrocortisone ointment 0.5–1% used sparingly
- Oral antihistamine, e.g. promethazine hydrochloride (Phenergan) 25–50 mg at night

Vagina

Vaginitis and vaginal discharge

The commonest disorder of the vagina is vaginitis – either infective or atrophic. These conditions and the differential diagnosis of vaginal discharge are discussed in Chapter 7. Atrophic vaginitis should be treated with local or systemic oestrogen.

Vaginal prolapse

For discussion of vaginal prolapse, see Chapter 21.

Box 17.3 Congenital disorders, cysts and tumours of the vagina

These are uncommon but include the following:

- Imperforate hymen
- Vaginal agenesis
- Complete or partial duplication of the vagina
- Vaginal adenosis
- Gärtner's duct cyst
- Endometriotic cyst
- Inclusion cyst
- Cyst of paraurethral glands
- Fibromyoma, lipoma, myxoma

Congenital disorders, cysts and tumours of the vagina

'Imperforate hymen'

- The occluding membrane is in fact not the hymen but results from failure of fusion of the müllerian portion of the vagina with that derived from the urogenital sinus.
- *Cryptomenorrhoea* – hidden menstruation.
- *Haematocolpos* – accumulation of menstrual blood in the vagina.
- *Hydrocolpos* – accumulation of mucoid fluid in the vagina in a neonate is a less common mode of presentation.
- Usually presents at around the age of 14 with primary amenorrhoea, intermittent lower abdominal pain at the time of (hidden) menstruation and often with retention of urine with or without overflow.
- Diagnosis is made by inspection of the vulva which usually reveals a bulging bluish membrane at the vaginal introitus. The haematocolpos may be palpable abdominally often with the distended bladder above it. A rectal examination, not always necessary, will confirm the presence of vaginal distension. Diagnosis can be confirmed by ultrasound but not normally necessary.
- Treatment is by incision of the occluding membrane, under general anaesthesia,

with release of chocolate-coloured old blood. In a patient with a single vagina the occluding membrane is usually the only abnormality.

Vaginal agenesis

- Partial vaginal agenesis may occur in the presence of a functioning uterus. The presentation will be the same as with an imperforate hymen but usually earlier. Treatment by vaginal construction.
- If the uterus is absent, an artificial vagina may be constructed if required or Williams' operation (formation of a perineal pouch by apposition of the labia majora) may be performed.

Complete or partial duplication of the vagina

- Complete duplication of the vagina is usually associated with a double cervix and double uterus and is usually asymptomatic and found during a routine vaginal examination. Treatment is not normally required.
- Partial duplication of the vagina in association with a double uterus may present with unilateral haematocolpos which eventually causes lower abdominal discomfort and retention of urine but not primary amenorrhoea. A concomitant renal abnormality is commonly found and an intravenous urogram should be performed.

Vaginal adenosis

- Patient's mother may have taken diethylstilboestrol in pregnancy.
- Areas of columnar epithelium in vagina.
- Structural abnormalities of vagina, cervix and uterus may be present as well.
- Malignant change may occur with development of vaginal carcinoma; therefore, requires close follow-up.

Gärtner's duct cyst

- Mesonephric remnant in anterolateral aspect of vagina.
- Usually asymptomatic and best left untreated unless causing a problem.

Endometriotic cyst

- Endometriosis in the pouch of Douglas may involve the posterior fornix of the vagina.
- Usually palpable nodularity rather than a visible cyst.
- Treatment usually medical rather than surgical.

Inclusion cyst

- Usually in lower posterior wall of vagina following childbirth or surgical procedures.

- Excise if necessary.

Cyst of paraurethral glands

- In lower anterior vaginal wall.
- If asymptomatic best left alone. If symptomatic refer to a urologist.

Fibromyoma, lipoma, myxoma etc.

These may occur and may require excision.

Cervix

Box 17.4 Non-malignant lesions of the cervix

- Cervical ectropion (Figure 17.1)
- Cervicitis
- Retention cysts
- Cervical polyp (Figure 17.1)
- Condylomata acuminata

Non-malignant lesions of the cervix

Cervical ectropion

- Squamocolumnar junction lies on ectocervix and columnar epithelium is therefore visible round external os (Figure 17.1).

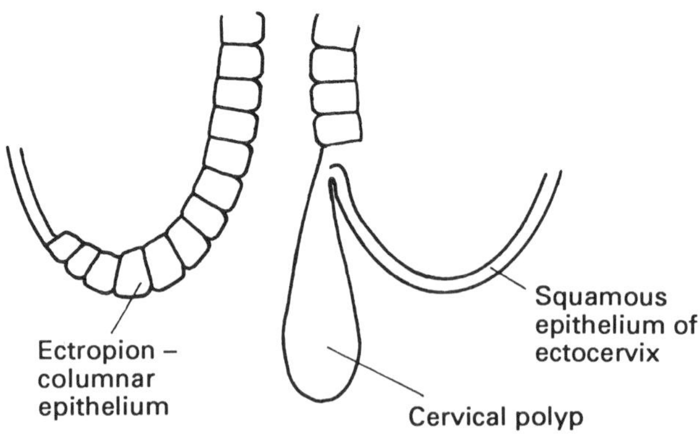

Figure 17.1 Diagrammatic representation of cervical ectropion and cervical polyp.

- Can occur in anyone in reproductive age group, but commonest when oestrogen levels are increased as in pregnancy and in those taking combined oral contraceptives.

- Columnar epithelium may also be visible in parous women as the cervix is often patulous.
- Usually asymptomatic but may cause discharge and postcoital bleeding.
- If asymptomatic no treatment required but patients should have regular smears (see Chapter 18).
- If causes symptoms and smear and/or colposcopy is normal cautery, cryocautery, diathermy or laser treatment may be performed (Box 17.5).

Box 17.5 Cervical cautery/cryocautery/diathermy/laser treatment

- Indicated for treatment of symptomatic cervical ectropion
- Patient should be warned that she will have increased discharge for a few weeks; should be advised not to have intercourse for 4–6 weeks
- The slough separates at about 10 days and there may be bleeding then; healing takes 4–6 weeks
- A course of intravaginal antibiotic (Sultrin) cream is often prescribed

Cervicitis

Inflammation of the cervix which may cause vaginal discharge.

- Acute cervicitis may be due to bacterial infection with *Neisseria gonorrhoeae* or *Chlamydia trachomatis* and is then usually part of a generalized acute pelvic inflammatory process or it may be due to viral infection with herpes or papilloma virus (see Chapter 7).
- Chronic cervicitis – endocervical canal is inflamed; specific organisms not usually identifiable. Treatment is with cautery, cryocautery, diathermy or laser.

Cervical retention cysts (nabothian follicles)

- Common in parous women.
- Caused by blockage of ducts of endocervical glands.
- Usually asymptomatic and no treatment required; can be destroyed by cautery, cryocautery, diathermy or laser.

Cervical polyp

- Pedunculated polyp usually arising from endocervical canal but may arise from endometrium and protrude through the cervix.
- If arises from the cervix is usually bright red and formed of adenomatous tissue with vascular stroma.
- Usually single but occasionally multiple.
- Often asymptomatic but can cause intermenstrual, postcoital or postmenopausal bleeding.

- Usually removed under anaesthetic by twisting the pedicle until polyp avulsed and then cauterizing the base. Dilatation and curettage should be performed at the same time to exclude intrauterine pathology if bleeding has occurred.

Condylomata acuminata (warts)

- Caused by human papilloma virus.
- Can occur on the cervix as well as on the vulva.
- Treatment as for vulval warts.

Chapter 18

Cervical, vaginal and vulval intraepithelial neoplasia

Invasive carcinoma of the cervix is preceded by pre-invasive changes which usually take place over several years. It is important to detect these changes so that relatively simple and effective treatment can be given to prevent the development of invasive cancer. For classification and management see Table 18.1.

Table 18.1 Classification and management of cervical intraepithelial neoplasia (CIN)

CIN classification	*WHO classification*	*Cytology*[a]	*Histology*[b]	*Management*
CIN I	Mild dysplasia	Cells have enlarged, irregular hyperchromatic nuclei and uneven chromatin distribution Multinucleation Plentiful cytoplasm	Abnormal cells occupy basal third of epithelium	Treat infection Repeat smear in 6 months and colposcope if CIN suspected; if negative repeat smear in 6 months and then yearly
CIN II	Moderate dysplasia	As for CIN I but nearly 50% of the cell is occupied by the nucleus	Abnormal cells occupy one- to two-thirds of epithelium	Colposcopy and biopsy before local treatment or cone biopsy; then repeat smear at 4 months, 10 months and then yearly (CIN II and CIN III)
CIN III	Severe dysplasia – carcinoma *in situ*	As for CIN II but more than 50% of the cell is occupied by the nucleus	Abnormal cells occupy full thickness of epithelium Many mitotic figures Lack of stratification	

[a]Diagnosis depends mainly on nuclear changes.
[b]Diagnosis depends mainly on proportion of epithelium occupied by abnormal cells.

- The *squamocolumnar junction* is the junction between the squamous epithelium of the ectocervix and the columnar epithelium of the endocervical canal.
- In postmenopausal women, the squamocolumnar junction often lies inside the cervical canal making it difficult to take an adequate smear unless a cytobrush (Figure 18.1) is used as well as a spatula.
- *Ectropion* – in women in the reproductive age group, particularly during pregnancy and in those taking the contraceptive pill, the squamocolumnar junction may be on

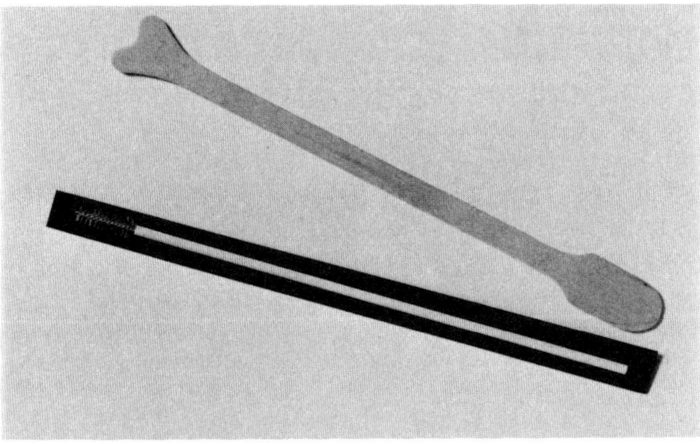

Figure 18.1 Ayre's spatula and cytobrush.

the ectocervix several millimetres from the external os giving the appearance on speculum examination previously known as an *erosion.*

- Exposure of endocervical columnar epithelium to the acidity of the vagina stimulates metaplasia into squamous epithelium. The area of metaplastic change is known as the *transformation zone.*
- Infections, particularly herpes simplex virus (type II) and human papilloma virus (type 6, 11, 16, 18), and possibly contact with other irritants, such as smegma, disturb normal metaplastic transformation and may promote dysplasia. These promoting factors are related to sexual activity, hence the association of dysplasia with early coital experience and multiple sexual partners.
- The term 'cervical intraepithelial neoplasia' (CIN) replaces the World Health Organisation (WHO) classification and CIN I, II and III equate with mild, moderate and severe dysplasia or carcinoma *in situ* (Table 18.1). Not all CIN lesions progress to invasive carcinoma. Progression to malignancy may take many years but can occur much more rapidly.
- Intraepithelial neoplastic change of the cervix can be detected with a smear (Box 18.1). The squamocolumnar junction and transformation zone are scraped with a wooden or plastic spatula (Figure 18.1) and the cells are spread onto a slide and fixed. When the squamocolumnar junction lies in the canal a specially shaped spatula and a cytobrush should be used.

Frequency of cervical cytological screening

An effective cytological screening programme fulfils the following requirements:

- Delivery to all women at risk.
- Repeated at optimal intervals.
- Close liaison between laboratory, medical staff and patients to ensure comprehensive cost effective service.

Box 18.1 Taking a smear

- Reassure the patient and explain the procedure to her
- With the patient in the dorsal or left lateral position introduce bivalve (Cusco's) speculum and locate cervix
- Select appropriate spatula, and cytobrush if necessary
- Apply spatula to cervix placing the longest part of the blade into the cervical canal; rotate 360° clockwise, and then anticlockwise to improve sampling
- Spread scrapings from both sides of spatula thinly onto a glass slide
- Fix smear immediately by spraying with ether or dipping into alcohol; cells rapidly become distorted if allowed to dry before fixing

Note

- Contamination by blood and discharge complicates interpretation considerably; do not take a smear during menstruation
- Ensure correct labelling of slides and cytology form
- In pregnancy the cervix is soft and vascular; take care not to provoke bleeding; if bleeding does occur reassure patient and give her a sanitary pad

Problems in the diagnosis of cervical carcinoma

- The majority of patients who develop invasive cervical carcinoma, particularly those over 40 years of age, have never had a smear.
- Approximately 10% of positive smears may not be associated with CIN when the cervix is examined colposcopically.
- Poor technique in smear taking and laboratory error contribute to screening failures – false negatives (Box 18.2).
- It has been suggested from one study that screening with appropriate intervention every 5 years would reduce the incidence of invasive cervical cancer by 84%, every 3 years by 91% and every year by 93%, but different figures have been suggested by other groups.

Box 18.2 Reasons for false negative smears

- Errors in taking the smear
- Presence of blood or exudate
- Smear applied too thinly or too thickly or allowed to dry before fixation
- Laboratory error
- Lesion is very small or entirely inside cervical canal

- A possible ideal, but currently usually impractical, approach for cervical screening would be to commence screening a few months after first coitus and to take a second smear 6–12 months later and another 1 year later if both early smears were normal. Smears would then be taken at 3-yearly intervals up to the age of 65 years if both partners had been and remained faithful. In other circumstances smears would need to be taken more often.
- The intercollegiate working party's recent recommendation was that all women between the ages of 20 and 64 should be invited to have a smear every 3 years and that there should be no upper age limit for women who have never had a smear.
- The actual programme followed will depend on local resources both in terms of finance and laboratory staff.
- All women should be made aware of the recommended screening intervals, and should be informed of their results. A computerized call/recall system minimizes slip ups.
- The quality of the screening programme should be closely monitored and someone of appropriate ability should supervise the organization of the service.
- Patients with abnormal smears should have easy access to prompt and appropriate management.

Colposcopy

A colposcope is a low power (× 5–40) binocular microscope used to examine changes on the surface of the cervix, vagina and vulva and to define the severity and extent of lesions.

- Important to reassure that often no treatment or only simple treatment will be necessary as many patients referred for colposcopy are unnecessarily anxious.
- Lithotomy position.
- Cusco's speculum introduced to allow visualization of cervix.
- Cervix cleaned gently with physiological saline to remove discharge and mucus. Examination through a green filter (optional) accentuates vascular patterns.
- Acetic acid (5%) is applied. Patient should be warned that she may feel a sensation of cold or 'stinging'. Proteins in dividing cells are denatured to produce opaque, white patches. Acetowhite epithelium is found where columnar epithelium is replaced by metaplastic squamous epithelium across the transformation zone; it is present where there is infection with human papilloma virus (HPV) and when there is CIN or invasive carcinoma. (Invasive carcinoma should, however, be detected on examination with the naked eye.) Where CIN is present the intercapillary distance is increased and terminal vessels of columnar villi are isolated by atypical epithelial growth to produce the topographic picture of punctate or mosaic patterns. The more coarse and well demarcated the appearance, the more likely is the lesion to be severe. Atypical terminal vessels are a feature of microinvasion or frank invasive carcinoma.

- When the upper limit of the lesion is clearly visualized, biopsies are taken from the most severely affected areas, after warning the patient.
- When the upper limit of the lesion is inside the cervical canal, cone biopsy is required for diagnosis and for treatment (Figure 18.3).
- If microinvasive disease (Chapter 20) is suspected cytologically and/or on colposcopy or histology, cone biopsy is mandatory.
- Some bleeding is likely following biopsy. This is readily controlled using a silver nitrate stick. Inform the patient that spotting is likely and provide a sanitary pad.
- The implications of the findings must be fully explained to the patient and an early date given for any necessary treatment.
- A small percentage of lesions extend onto the fornices.

Cervicography

This is a new technique in which close-up photographs of the cervix are taken with a hand-held camera before and after treatment of the cervix with acetic acid. The photographs can be taken by paramedical staff and are then interpreted by an expert colposcopist. The technique is being evaluated as the waiting lists for colposcopy are so long; currently the false positive rates are high.

Treatment

Local treatment is feasible when the entire lesion is visualized and CIN is confirmed histologically. Abnormal epithelium is destroyed allowing replacement by healthy squamous epithelium.

- Cryocautery, 'cold' coagulation (actually 100°C), deep needle diathermy and carbon dioxide laser are all used to destroy affected epithelium. Because there may be abnormal epithelium in endocervical gland crypts, the destructive ability of any method used should reach a depth of 5–7 mm.
- The cure rate with all modalities is of the order of 90–95%.
- During pregnancy the cervix is soft and vascular. Unless the lesion looks suspicious of invasive carcinoma, the cervix is examined colposcopically every 3 months and treatment is deferred until 3 months postnatally.

Cryocautery (Figure 18.2)

The most appropriate probe for the contour of the cervix is chosen; a cycle of freeze (using nitrous oxide or carbon dioxide), defreeze and refreeze of the order of 2–3 minutes on, 2–5 minutes off and 2–3 minutes on is usual but will vary from one operator to another. Timing starts when the ice ball around the probe reaches 4 mm.

- No anaesthetic required.
- Destruction is only to a depth of 4 mm.
- Cramp-like discomfort is felt by many women.
- Copious vaginal discharge follows treatment.

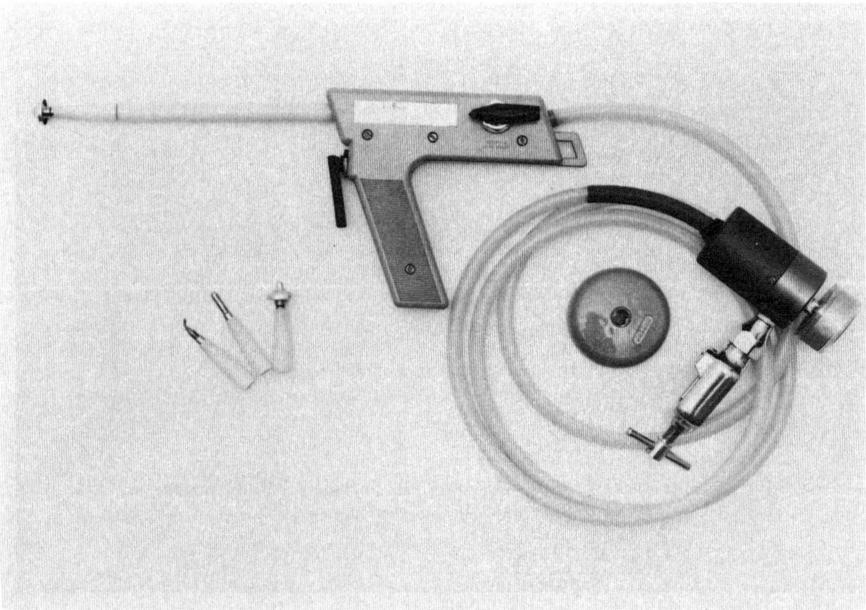

Figure 18.2 Cryocautery.

- Failure is likely with large lesions and if cervix is scarred leading to poor cryoprobe contact.
- Retraction of the new squamocolumnar junction into the cervical canal may occur.

'Cold' coagulation

Appropriate thermal probes are selected and heat, usually around 100°C, is used for treatment. Abnormal epithelium is destroyed by 20 second application of the probe to affected areas.

- No anaesthetic required.
- Destruction only reaches 3–4 mm.
- Cramp-like discomfort may be experienced.
- Vaginal discharge and bleeding may occur.

Electrodiathermy (deep needle diathermy)

Lesion is defined colposcopically or delineated by application of iodine. A needle electrode with coagulator setting at about 4 is used to a depth of 5–7 mm thus ensuring destruction of affected epithelium which includes the deep gland crypts. A ball electrode can then be traced over the lesion and into the endocervical canal to complete ablation.

- General or regional anaesthesia required.

- Complications such as infection, secondary bleeding and cervical stenosis occur in about 3% of cases.

Laser

Carbon dioxide lasers are usually used to produce an invisible infrared beam of 10 μm wavelength focused to a diameter of 2 mm at point of contact. The laser is attached to a colposcope and manipulated to provide colposcopically directed, precise destruction of abnormal epithelium to the required depth of 5–7 mm. Intermittent predetermined bursts or a continuous beam are used for ablation therapy.

- Acceptable to many patients as an outpatient procedure without anaesthesia; paracervical block is used if necessary.
- Cramp-like discomfort and a pin-prick or burning feeling is experienced by most women.
- Troublesome bleeding occurs in 1–2% of cases.
- Healing is rapid. Metaplastic cells cover the surface in 10 days and by 4 weeks the area is replaced by mature squamous epithelium.
- Minimal postoperative discharge or fibrosis.
- Vaginal extension of CIN can be treated under anaesthesia. Vaporization is adjusted to an appropriate depth.

Management after local destructive therapy

- A course of intravaginal antibiotic cream, such as Sultrin cream, is often prescribed.
- Discharge, lasting from a few days to 3–4 weeks, is likely.
- Spotting may occasionally be experienced 7–10 days after treatment. Advise patient to report to her doctor if bleeding is heavy. Exclude onset of menstruation.
- No coitus or tampons until after review in 6 weeks.
- Repeat cervical smear 4 months and 10 months after treatment and then yearly if normal.

Treatment

For treatment of cervical or vaginal HPV infections, see Box 18.3.

Box 18.3 Treatment of cervical or vaginal human papilloma virus infections

- Cervical HPV can be treated by all the above forms of local destructive therapy
- Most resistant or recurrent cervical HPV infections respond to two or three applications of 5-fluorouracil; great care required, avoid contact with vulva as very painful
- Vaginal HPV also responds well to one or two applications of 5-fluorouracil
- Treatment can be repeated at 7- to 10-day intervals

Cone biopsy

Cone biopsy (Figure 18.3) is required when the upper limit of abnormal epithelium is inside the endocervical canal and cannot be visualized using the colposcope. It may also be required when the colposcopic appearance is suspicious but not diagnostic of microinvasive or invasive carcinoma.

- Performed in approximately 25% of patients with CIN.
- General or regional anaesthesia required.
- Outer limit of lesion defined by colposcopy or by application of Lugol's iodine (Schiller's test). Abnormal epithelium produces little or no glycogen and will not stain dark brown.
- An intracervical injection of pitressin 20 units in 20 ml saline, or of adrenaline 1:200 000, will reduce bleeding and can be given if there are no contraindications, after consultation with the anaesthetist.
- Haemostatic sutures may be placed at 3 and 9 o'clock to catch the descending cervical vessels.
- A circular cut is made with cold knife or laser. The cut is directed parallel to and then towards the cervical canal to a predetermined depth (see Figure 18.3).
- Further stitches can be inserted to secure haemostasis in large cone biopsies.
- Ensure patency of cervical canal by passage of 8 mm dilator.
- With small cones, Oxycel may aid haemostasis.
- A pack and catheter may be inserted for 24 hours.
- Biopsy specimen is marked with a stitch at 12 o'clock for orientation by histopathologist.

Subsequent management

- Primary haemorrhage occurs in a small percentage of patients. Close observation after surgery is required.

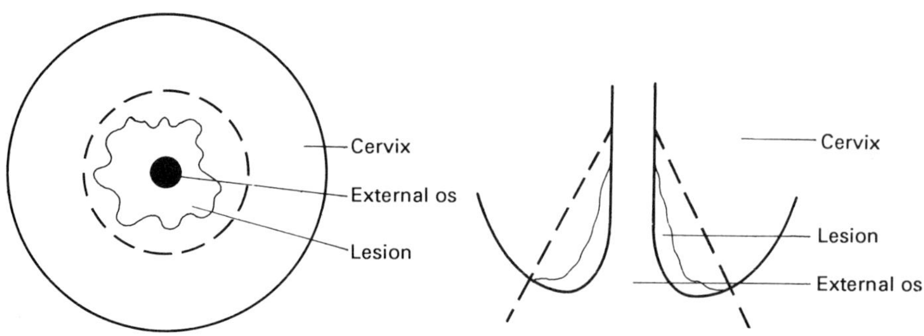

Figure 18.3 Cone biopsy.

- Patient must be warned of possibility (5–10%) of secondary haemorrhage 10–21 days after surgery.
- Review 6 weeks after surgery.
- Cone biopsy is adequate treatment for CIN and usually for microinvasion if margins are clear of disease (see Chapter 20).
- Invasive carcinoma requires radical hysterectomy (Wertheim's hysterectomy) or radiotherapy (see Chapter 20).
- Further colposcopy and biopsy followed by local destructive therapy may suffice for incomplete excision of CIN at ectocervical margin. Repeat cone biopsy or hysterectomy will be necessary for incomplete excision at endocervical margin if cytology remains abnormal; this should be performed 4 months after original surgery when inflammatory changes will have subsided. Repeated diagnostic endocervical curettage may be an option when fertility is of paramount importance.
- Subfertility due to poor mucus production may follow cone biopsy in a small percentage of cases.
- A large cone may cause cervical incompetence if the internal os is damaged.
- Cervical stenosis occurs after a small percentage of cone biopsies – most commonly following the removal of a long (more than 2 cm) cone of tissue. Complete occlusion of the canal results in amenorrhoea, and lower abdominal pain at the time of the missed periods. Stenosis of the canal can cause dysmenorrhoea and can lead to failure of the cervix to dilate in labour – if this is not recognized it may lead to rupture of the uterus.
- Repeat smear 4 and 10 months after cone biopsy and then yearly if normal.
- When adenocarcinoma *in situ* (AIS) or glandular atypia is diagnosed, 4-monthly smears with a spatula and endocervical cytobrush for 2 years followed by yearly smears are advised if excision margins are clear. Hysterectomy 4 months after original cone biopsy is currently recommended when margins of excision are not clear of disease (Box 18.4), but the optimum management of this condition has not yet been established.

Box 18.4 Incomplete margin of excision

- Found in an appreciable number of cone biopsy specimens
- Incomplete endocervical margin gives most cause for concern; incomplete ectocervical margin is easy to re-examine and treat
- Local treatment can be given for detectable residual non-invasive disease
- Follow-up is imperative
- Microinvasive disease can be treated by repeat cone biopsy or simple hysterectomy
- Radical surgery or radiotherapy is necessary when invasive disease is present

Vaginal intraepithelial neoplasia (VAIN)

- Pre-invasive and microinvasive lesions in the vagina are uncommon; they are mainly found in the upper third of the vagina.
- Some 4% of cervical lesions extend onto the vagina.
- Some 0.2–8% of patients develop VAIN within 10–15 years of hysterectomy for CIN hence the need for follow-up vault smears for cytology.
- The lesions are usually asymptomatic.
- Colposcopic appearances are similar to those in the cervix and an association with HPV is often found.

Management

- Colposcopy should always include inspection of the upper vagina.
- Biopsy followed by local destructive therapy or excision is required when VAIN is detected.
- Where hysterectomy is considered necessary for other reasons in a patient with VAIN, a vaginal cuff is taken to include the lesions (defined by Schiller's test). Vaginal hysterectomy is particularly suitable.
- After hysterectomy for CIN, vault smears using the rounded end of the Ayre's spatula should be taken at 4 months and 10 months and then yearly if normal.
- One or two applications of 5-fluorouracil are effective against more than 95% of HPV infections; great care is required with this form of treatment.

Vulval intraepithelial neoplasia (VIN)

These lesions appear to be on the increase with a likelihood that they are sexually transmitted and associated with a long (10 years or more) history of infection, particularly with HPV. They tend to be multifocal and often coexist with intraepithelial lesions in the vagina and cervix. Atypical or dystrophic vulval lesions are either hypoplastic or hyperplastic or mixed (see Chapter 17).

- Lesions are usually multifocal, well demarcated, flat or raised and white or pink.
- May be asymptomatic but 80% of patients experience pruritus and soreness.
- Colposcopy is increasingly being used to detect abnormal areas and to direct biopsy. Pre-treatment of the cleansed vulva with a 1% aqueous solution of toluidine blue followed after 2 minutes by a wash with 1% aqueous acetic acid will stain parakeratotic areas blue.
- VIN requires definitive treatment by excision or laser ablation; following laser ablation the treated area heals in 6 weeks.

Chapter 19

Pelvic mass

- There are several organs in the pelvis which can enlarge, distend or produce cysts.
- The pelvis is reasonably capacious, and so a mass may not be noticed until it rises above the pelvic brim or produces other symptoms
- Although the patient may notice the mass or present with symptoms due to it, many lesions are first detected on routine pelvic examination at Family Planning or Well Woman Clinics, or during ultrasound or occasionally X-ray examination of the pelvis.
- Once a pelvic mass is detected, every effort must be made to make a diagnosis.

History

Important points are:

- Duration of awareness of the mass.
- Rate of growth.
- Presence, type and onset of any symptoms.
- General health, changes in weight and alterations in bowel and bladder function.
- Alterations in menstrual cycle and presence or absence of dyspareunia.

General examination

- Assess the patient as a whole for evidence of weight loss, anaemia or hormonal abnormalities such as hirsutism.
- Inspect the abdomen for evidence of distension, peristalsis, scars, pigmentation, size and shape of any mass arising from the pelvis.
- Palpate the left and right hypochondrial quadrants before the lower abdomen. Demonstrate that the mass is arising from the pelvis by failure to get below it. Register the presence of tenderness and hyperaesthesia. Use percussion to identify gaseous distension and check for the presence of ascites.
- Note the size and shape, the position and mobility, and the regularity and consistency of the mass.

Vaginal examination

This must be preceded by general and abdominal examination:

- *Vulva* – look for any abnormality including clitoral enlargement, vulval tumours or ulceration, signs of infection, varicosities, obvious prolapse or perineal deficiency.
- *Vagina* – using speculum look for discharge, vaginitis, prolapse or any other abnormality.
- *Cervix* – assess normality and position and note any bleeding or discharge through the cervical os.
- *Bimanual palpation* – systematically examine to ascertain the size, position and consistency of the mass. Is the uterus enlarged or displaced? Is the mass separate from the uterus? Does palpation cause pain? Is there any pain on moving the cervix? – cervical excitation pain.

Pregnancy

- History is usually helpful. Uterus is central, symmetrically enlarged and soft.
- Ectopic pregnancy can produce a pelvic mass in the ampulla or by haematoma formation.

Fibroids (uterine leiomyomas)

- Common uterine tumours occurring in approximately one in five women particularly between 35 and 50 years of age.
- Vary in diameter from 1–2 mm to 10 cm or more.
- Usually multiple.
- More common in Negroid women
- Oestrogen promotes growth and they tend to regress or become calcified following the menopause.

Clinical considerations

- Fibroids may be subserous, intramural, submucous, polypoid or cervical (Figure 19.1).
- Often asymptomatic.
- When vascular supply is compromised, particularly in pregnancy, ischaemic necrosis or red degeneration occurs causing pain. Hyaline or cystic degeneration or calcification may follow.
- Sarcomatous change occurs in less than 0.5% of fibroids.
- *Subserous* – commonly enlarge to form an obvious pelvic mass and may cause pressure symptoms; often pedunculated, rarely undergo torsion with resultant pain; can extend into the broad ligament; rarely become attached secondarily to surrounding organs in parasitic fashion. A rare complication is ascites and pleural effusion (pseudo-Meigs' syndrome).

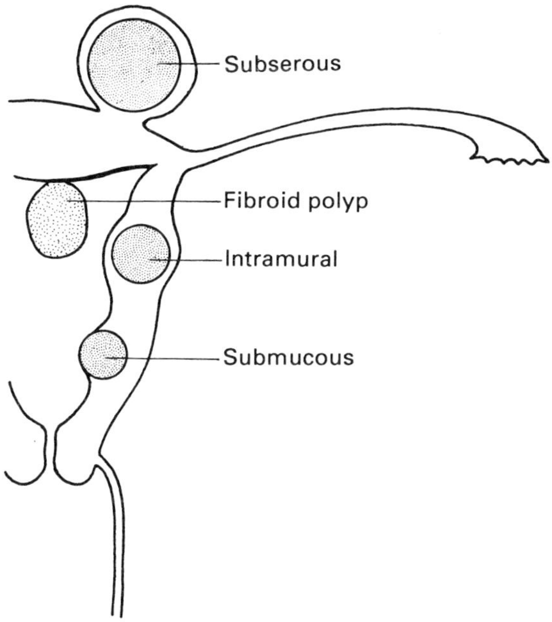

Figure 19.1 Diagrammatic representation of some possible sites of fibroids. (From *Miscarriage. The Facts*, G. Lachelin, 1985, Figure 8.3, Oxford University Press, by permission).

- *Intramural* – enlargement produces a pelvic mass which can press on neighbouring organs, become impacted and may rarely produce urinary retention. Increased vascularity and enlargement of the uterine cavity may cause menorrhagia.
- *Submucous* – increase the size of the uterine cavity and cause menorrhagia. Fertility may be impaired.
- *Fibroid polyp* – may cause menorrhagia or intermenstrual bleeding or colicky pain as uterus attempts to expel it. A fundal fibroid polyp can cause uterine inversion (see Chapter 21).
- *Cervical* – cause distortion of the cervix.
- Role in subfertility and miscarriage often difficult to determine. Many women with fibroids have successful pregnancies but a submucous fibroid or polyp obviously can cause problems.

Diagnosis

- Palpation.
- Ultrasound to confirm the diagnosis and to exclude ovarian abnormality.
- Hysterosalpingogram will demonstrate submucous fibroids, or a fibroid polyp.
- May be first noticed at time of D and C or hysteroscopy.
- Direct observation by laparoscopy or at laparotomy.

Expectant management

Small (5 cm or less) asymptomatic fibroids require explanation and reassurance and review at intervals. Fibroids with minimal symptoms, detected at the perimenopause, may be managed conservatively by awaiting the menopause and probable atrophy, provided the diagnosis is certain and an ovarian tumour has been excluded.

Medical treatment

- Includes iron therapy to treat or avert anaemia.
- LHRH analogues may be used to reduce the size of fibroids but cause severe menopausal symptoms and the fibroids revert to their previous size after treatment. Can be used as a temporary measure.

Surgical treatment

- Indicated for fibroid polyp – via cervix if cervix dilated, or by hysterotomy if no cervical dilatation.
- Required when symptoms are troublesome, or there is concern about possible sarcomatous change.

Myomectomy

- Considered when preservation of the uterus, particularly for reproductive function, is required. Patient should be told that uncontrollable bleeding may rarely necessitate hysterectomy.
- Caesarean section may be indicated in a subsequent pregnancy if the uterine cavity is entered.
- A major problem is the likely development of further fibroids.
- Adhesion formation is not uncommon following myomectomy.

Hysterectomy

- Performed when preservation of the uterus is not required or when myomectomy is not possible.

Ovarian cysts

Ovarian cysts contain fluid or semisolid material. They may be unilocular or multilocular and it may be impossible to determine whether they are benign or malignant by macroscopic inspection.

Follicular cysts

- Formed by the action of follicle stimulating hormone (FSH) on ovarian follicles in one or both ovaries. Persist if ovulation does not ensue.

- Most common in the perimenopause or if there are adhesions round the ovary or following ovarian stimulation with exogenous gonadotrophins.
- Not usually more than 5 cm in diameter.
- Continued oestrogen production disrupts the normal cycle.
- Shortened or lengthened menstrual cycle or irregular vaginal bleeding may occur.
- Occasionally cause discomfort or undergo torsion or even rupture.
- Usually resolve spontaneously within 6–8 weeks. If fail to resolve may be aspirated under ultrasound or laparoscopic guidance. The fluid must be examined cytologically and the patient must be reviewed after 4 weeks to ensure that the cyst is not re-forming.

Corpus luteum cyst

- Rarely occurs unless the woman is pregnant.
- May be up to 5 cm diameter.
- Usually asymptomatic.
- May cause discomfort, or even undergo torsion or rupture.
- Management is conservative unless undergoes complications.

Theca lutein cysts

- Follow stimulation by high levels of chorionic gonadotrophin from hydatidiform mole or choriocarcinoma, or excessive dosage of drugs used in induction of ovulation.
- Altered bleeding pattern, discomfort, torsion or rupture may occur.
- May be associated with hyperstimulation syndrome of varying degrees of severity including multilocular cyst formation, ascites and hypovolaemic shock.
- Usually resolve after HCG stimulation ceases.
- Admission for rest, rehydration and analgesia is necessary when the hyperstimulation syndrome occurs.

Dermoid cyst

- Often found inadvertently during routine examination.
- Bilateral in approximately 20% of cases.
- Ectodermal, mesodermal and endodermal elements may all be present.

Symptoms

- Usually asymptomatic, but pressure symptoms and pain associated with torsion may occur.

Management

- Ovarian cystectomy; the other ovary must always be checked.

Serous cystadenoma

- Usually unilocular and often bilateral.
- Lined by ciliated columnar epithelium with tendency to formation of papilliferous projections and production of straw-coloured fluid.

Mucinous cystadenoma

- Usually large multiloculated cyst.
- Lined by columnar cells secreting mucinous material.
- Bilateral in approximately 10% of cases.
- Spillage of mucinous material into peritoneal cavity may result in condition called pseudomyxoma peritonei.

Endometriotic cystadenoma

Lining of cyst resembles that of the endometrium. Usually filled with chocolate-coloured altered blood; found in association with endometriosis (see Chapter 8).

Symptoms caused by cystadenoma

- Symptoms from pressure on bowel or bladder, or pain if the cyst ruptures or torsion occurs.
- Endometriotic cyst may present with dysmenorrhoea.

Management of cystadenoma

- Ovarian cystectomy in the young, oophorectomy in the older woman. Always check other ovary for pathology.

Benign solid ovarian tumours

These are ovarian epithelial tumours with varying stromal content (adenofibroma) or cyst formation (cystadenofibroma). Functional tumours may be feminizing (granulosa or theca cell tumour) or virilizing (hilar cell or arrhenoblastoma).

Symptoms

- Fibromas very rarely produce ascites and hydrothorax (Meigs' syndrome).
- Functional effects such as hirsutism may be evident; bleeding pattern may be altered.

Management

- Laparotomy and oophorectomy with exploration of contralateral ovary are required. Careful histological examination is mandatory as some of these tumours are malignant.

Tubal mass

- This may be a hydrosalpinx or tubo-ovarian inflammatory mass (or an ectopic pregnancy, or carcinoma of the fallopian tube – very rare).
- There may or may not be a history of overt infection.
- The condition may be bilateral.

Symptoms

- Pelvic discomfort, dyspareunia, subfertility, menorrhagia and dysmenorrhoea.

Management

- In the quiescent stage, conservative management may be appropriate.
- Cuff salpingostomy may be required to attempt to enhance fertility when a hydrosalpinx is detected, but the success rate is usually less than 10% and there is an increased risk of ectopic pregnancy.
- Unilateral or bilateral salpingo-oophorectomy with or without hysterectomy may be a last resort for treatment of recurrent chronic debilitating pelvic pain.

Pelvic mass due to neoplasia of the genital tract

For this see Chapter 21.

Non-gynaecological causes of pelvic mass

- The bladder, sigmoid colon and rectum are the main non-genital pelvic organs.

Urinary tract

- A distended bladder causes a pelvic mass. It is essential to ask a patient to empty her bladder before performing a vaginal examination. Any residual bladder distension will then be due to retention.

- An ectopic kidney is a rare cause of a pelvic mass.

Gynaecological causes of urinary retention

- An impacted retroverted gravid uterus (at about 14–16 weeks' gestation).
- Impaction of an ovarian cyst or fibroid uterus in the pelvis.
- Procidentia producing acute angulation of the urethra and obstruction to flow.
- Haematocolpos (see Chapter 17).

Alimentary tract

- The distended caecum can be mistaken for an ovarian cyst.
- Diverticulosis, faecal impaction and neoplasia can all produce a pelvic mass.

Pelvic mass – diagnosis

- If the clinical assessment suggests a pelvic mass whose nature is uncertain, further investigation may be needed to assist diagnosis.

Non-invasive

- Ultrasound scanning is an increasingly effective means of assessing the nature of a pelvic mass.
- Magnetic resonance imaging is in its infancy but shows great promise and will probably become a valuable diagnostic adjunct.
- Radiology may be helpful in the diagnosis of abnormalities of the bowel or urinary tract.

Invasive

- Laparoscopy – macroscopic diagnosis can be made by direct vision.
- A simple ovarian cyst can be aspirated; this approach is not suitable with a large cyst. The fluid must be sent for cytological examination.
- Laparotomy may be indicated when laparoscopy is contraindicated or when surgical treatment is required.

Management

For the management of a patient with a pelvic mass see Box 19.1.

Box 19.1 Management of a patient with a pelvic mass

- The patient is understandably anxious and may be worried that the mass is malignant
- Discuss with her the probable diagnosis and, if you don't think that it is malignant, reassure her
- Explain the diagnostic steps involved
- Discuss the probable management
- Explain fully the consequence of any treatment that may be necessary

Chapter 20

Genital carcinoma

Twenty per cent of women in developed countries die from cancer; 20% of these deaths are due to breast cancer and 14% are due to genital cancer – most commonly ovarian, followed by cervical, endometrial and vulval cancer. Primary cancer of the fallopian tube and of the vagina are rare. For management of patients with cancer, see Box 20.1.

Box 20.1 Management of patient with cancer

Pre-treatment

- Patient will be understandably anxious
- Explanation of diagnosis and management must be unhurried and appropriate to the patient and her condition and all her questions must be answered
- Relatives must be involved if possible at an early stage and must be given sympathetic explanation and support; GP must be informed of management plan

Post-treatment

- Continuing support of patient and relatives will be required from hospital staff, GP and others as appropriate
- Long-term follow-up will entail check-ups at least every 3 or 4 months for 2 years; then every 6 months for a further 3 years and then yearly for at least another 5 years
- When all is found to be well the patient should be reassured and encouraged
- If a recurrence is detected further treatment should be fully discussed with the patient and arranged without delay
- The terminally ill patient will require much compassion and support, and suitable nursing care; pain relief should be appropriately chosen to allow her to be reasonably comfortable without being oversedated

Carcinoma of the vulva

Presentation

- Patient is usually over 60 years of age but carcinoma of the vulva also occurs in younger women in the 30- to 50-year-old age group. May follow a recognizable pre-invasive lesion.
- May present as an ulcer, as a raised lesion or as a fungating mass, usually in the anterior part of the vulva.
- Arises in the labia in approximately 85% of cases.
- May be unilateral or bilateral.

- Often presents late.
- Inguinal nodes are likely to be palpable if the lesion exceeds 4 cm diameter.
- Bilateral inguinal node involvement occurs in about 10% of cases.

Incidence

- Approximately 500 deaths in England and Wales per year.

Aetiology

- Vulval dystrophy is present in approximately 50% of cases.
- Especially in younger women there may be previous infection of the genital tract with human papilloma virus and there may be associated cervical and vaginal pre-invasive lesions.

Histology and pathology

- Biopsy is necessary to confirm the diagnosis.
- More than 90% of vulval carcinomas are squamous cell carcinomas.
- Spread is local and via lymphatics to inguinal, femoral and iliac lymph nodes (Box 20.2).
- Other vulval malignancies include melanoma, basal cell carcinoma, adenocarcinoma of Bartholin's glands, sarcoma and secondary carcinoma.
- Overall 5-year survival of carcinoma of the vulva following treatment is approximately 40%. The 5-year survival is approximately 70% if the nodes are not involved.

Box 20.2 Clinical staging of carcinoma of vulva

Stage I	2 cm or less in diameter and confined to vulva; nodes not palpable, or if palpable in either groin, mobile
Stage II	as for Stage I but more than 2 cm in diameter
Stage III	growth of any size with spread to urethra and/or vagina, perineum or anus with or without firm palpable nodes
Stage IV	involves upper urethral, bladder or rectal mucosa with or without fixity to bone; or distant metastases or ulcerated groin nodes are present

Management

- Full general and local examination.
- Biopsy the lesion.
- Assess suitability of surgical treatment. This will depend on stage of the disease and the patient's general condition. In an advanced case, palliative treatment may be all that is possible.
- If surgery is contemplated, ensure that patient is as fit for surgery as possible.

- Surgical treatment involves radical vulvectomy and bilateral groin dissection either at the same time or as a two-stage procedure.
- Explain fully to the patient and her relatives what surgery entails and the reasons for it. Vulvectomy is a particularly distressing operation and the patient is likely to be in hospital for several weeks.
- Radiotherapy is not usually used for primary treatment but can be helpful for treatment of recurrence.
- Chemotherapy is of little value.

Postoperative care

- An indwelling catheter is normally left in place for several days.
- Thromboembolism is a particular danger and physiotherapy is very important.
- Breakdown of wounds is not uncommon and occasionally skin grafting is required.

Subsequent management

- Local recurrence is commonest on the vulva but may occur in the groin if the nodes were affected. Treatment is with surgery and/or radiotherapy.
- Postoperative sequelae include urinary incontinence, vaginal prolapse and poor lymphatic drainage from the legs leading to lymphoedema.

Carcinoma of the vagina

Presentation

- Rare condition.
- Patient is usually over 60 years of age but carcinoma of the vagina also occurs in younger women exposed to specific aetiological factors.
- Primary lesions are less common than secondary spread from the genitourinary tract.
- May be associated with pre-invasive cervical, vaginal or vulval lesions.
- Usually presents with vaginal bleeding or blood-stained discharge.
- Examination may reveal an ulcerated or fungating lesion.
- Inguinal nodes may be palpable.
- In the case of secondary deposits in the vagina, symptoms from the primary lesion will usually, but not always, be present. Choriocarcinoma and hypernephroma occasionally present with vaginal secondaries.

Aetiology

- May be subsequent to chronic irritation as with a neglected ring pessary.

- May occur in relation to a general field change in the lower genital tract in association with pre-invasive or invasive disease of the cervix and vulva.
- Has been found to occur in association with vaginal adenosis in some of the daughters of women who were treated with diethylstilboestrol in pregnancy (Box 20.3).

Box 20.3 Vaginal adenosis

- Uncommon condition
- Has been found in the young adult daughters of women treated with diethylstilboestrol in pregnancy (mainly in the 1950s)
- There may be associated malformation of the genital tract
- Malignant change (clear cell adenocarcinoma) may occur and may cause irregular bleeding or blood-stained discharge

Histology and pathology

- Biopsy is necessary to make a diagnosis. More than 90% of primary vaginal carcinomas are of squamous origin but those arising in relation to exposure *in utero* to diethylstilboestrol are adenocarcinomas. Spread is via lymphatics, the lower third of the vagina draining to the inguinal nodes and the upper two-thirds to the pelvic nodes (Box 20.4).
- Overall 5-year survival following treatment is approximately 35%.

Box 20.4 Clinical staging of carcinoma of vagina

Stage I	confined to vaginal wall
Stage II	involves subvaginal tissue
Stage III	extends to pelvic wall
Stage IV	extends outside pelvis and/or involves bladder or rectal mucosa

Management

- Full general and local examination.
- Biopsy the lesion.
- Treatment will depend on the stage of the disease, the histology of the lesion and the age of the patient. Treatment is mainly with radiotherapy.

Carcinoma of the cervix

Presentation

- Patient is usually between 40 and 55 years of age but may be in younger or older age group.

- Presenting symptoms include postcoital, intermenstrual or postmenopausal bleeding or blood-stained discharge.
- Pain and urinary symptoms are late features of the disease. The ureters may be blocked off or a urinary fistula may occur.
- The cervix may be ulcerated or the lesion may be polypoidal. It may appear normal if there is an adenocarcinoma in the canal but the cervix will then usually be very firm and barrel shaped.
- There may be lateral or downward spread of the lesion.

Incidence

- Approximately 4000 new cases in England and Wales per year.
- Approximately 2000 deaths in England and Wales per year.

Aetiology

- Incidence increased in those who commence sexual activity at an early age and/or who have multiple partners, or whose partners have had multiple partners.
- Pre-invasive lesion commonly precedes development of invasive carcinoma.
- Human papilloma virus (especially type 16) infection may be an aetiological factor.

Histology and pathology

- Biopsy of the lesion is necessary to confirm the diagnosis.
- Approximately 90% are squamous carcinomas and the rest are mainly adenocarcinomas.
- Spread is local and via the lymphatics to pelvic nodes. Distant metastases are uncommon but may occur in the lungs, liver and bones and in the supraclavicular nodes (Box 20.5).

Box 20.5 Clinical staging of carcinoma of cervix

Stage I	confined to cervix	*Ia*	microinvasive carcinoma
		Ib	all other stage I
Stage II	extends beyond cervix but not to pelvic wall or to lower one-third of vagina	*IIa*	parametrium not involved
		IIb	parametrium involved
Stage III	extends to pelvic wall or lower one-third of vagina	*IIIa*	involves lower one-third of vagina but not pelvic wall
		IIIb	extends to pelvic wall and/or renal tract compromised
Stage IV	extends beyond true pelvis and/or involves bladder or rectal mucosa	*IVa*	involves adjacent organs
		IVb	involves distant organs

Notes staging disregards extension to corpus
inflammatory induration can confuse assessment of lateral spread

- The commonest causes of death are uraemia, infection and haemorrhage.
- The 5-year survival following treatment is approximately 85% for stage I, 70% for stage IIa, 55% for stage IIb, less than 30% for stage III and less than 10% for stage IV.

Management

- Full general, and vaginal and rectal examination.
- Full blood count, urea and electrolytes and liver function tests.
- Chest X-ray and intravenous urogram.
- Stage and biopsy the lesion; perform cystoscopy.
- Choice of treatment depends on stage of disease, age and fitness of patient and on the patient's informed choice.

Stage Ia (microinvasive carcinoma)

- Malignant cells breach the basement membrane with non-confluent invasion to a depth of less than 3–5 mm and a volume of less than 500 mm^3, and lymphatics and blood vessels are not involved (exact definition is variable at the present time).
- In a young woman, an adequate cone biopsy and continued surveillance as for pre-invasive lesions (see Chapter 18) is acceptable but pelvic nodes are involved in approximately 1% of cases.
- In an older woman, hysterectomy with assessment of pelvic nodes is preferable with continued follow-up.

Stage Ib and IIa

- Choice of therapy is between radical hysterectomy and radiotherapy. Small lesions are less likely to have lymph node involvement.

Surgery

- Preferable for younger women as it allows continued ovarian and coital function.
- Indicated when tumour is not radiosensitive or when there is associated uterine or ovarian pathology.
- The operation performed is a Wertheim's hysterectomy which entails removal of the uterus and cervix, the upper part of the vagina, the parametrium and pelvic lymph nodes.
- The bladder and ureters are especially vulnerable in a radical hysterectomy and postoperative bladder dysfunction is common.

Radiotherapy

- Used in stage I and IIa when patient not fit for surgery or in older woman when ovarian and coital function may not be important.
- Used for stages IIb, III and IV.
- Treatment is with a caesium source in the uterus and in the lateral vaginal fornices (usually two applications), followed by external radiotherapy to the pelvic walls.
- Complications of radiotherapy include nausea, lethargy and oestrogen-withdrawal symptoms, cystitis, proctitis, vaginitis and vaginal stenosis.

Chemotherapy

- Treatment with chemotherapy for cervical carcinoma is being developed and has been helpful in some cases.

Subsequent management

- Long-term follow-up is required with general and vaginal examination and cytology.
- Patients should be seen 3-monthly in the first year with particular attention being paid to the supraclavicular nodes and the abdomen and pelvis. Full blood count, urea and electrolytes and liver function tests are performed. Chest X-ray is performed every 2 years or more often if patient is symptomatic.
- Approximately 50% of patients who develop recurrence will do so in the first year, 70% by the end of the second year and 90% by the end of the fifth year.
- Pelvic exenteration may occasionally be appropriate for carefully selected patients with a central recurrence.
- Chemotherapy is occasionally of value for recurrent disease.

Pregnancy and cervical carcinoma

- This occurs in less than 0.5% of cases of cervical carcinoma.
- Adequate treatment of the carcinoma will entail termination of the pregnancy.

Carcinoma of the endometrium

Presentation

- Patient is usually in 50- to 70-year-old age group, but carcinoma of the endometrium may occur in younger or older age group (approximately 25% of patients are premenopausal or perimenopausal).
- Approximately 25% of patients are nulliparous.
- Presenting symptoms include postmenopausal or intermenstrual bleeding or discharge and menorrhagia.
- General and vaginal examination normally reveal no abnormality except in late

disease or if there is an associated abnormality such as fibroids or an ovarian tumour.

Incidence

- Approximately 3500 new cases in England and Wales per year.
- Approximately 1000 deaths in England and Wales per year.

Aetiology

- There is an association with nulliparity and with a late menopause.
- Associated with conditions that give rise to high levels of unopposed oestrogen, e.g. anovulation associated with polycystic ovary syndrome, exogenous oestrogen administration (without cyclical progestogen) and oestrogen-secreting tumours.
- Obesity leads to increased free oestrogen levels because of increased peripheral conversion of androgen to oestrogen in the fat and because sex hormone-binding globulin levels are lower in obese women.
- There may be a family history of endometrial carcinoma.

Histology and pathology

- Diagnosis is made by histological examination of endometrial curettings obtained by fractional curettage.
- Often preceded by atypical hyperplasia.
- Usually adenocarcinoma; rarely squamous or mixed tumour.
- Spread is by local infiltration and via lymphatics along uterine and ovarian vessels and round ligaments to pelvic, para-aortic and inguinal nodes. Lymphatic involvement occurs in about 10% of cases that are clinically stage I (Box 20.6).
- Ovarian secondaries are present in about 5% of cases that are clinically stage I.
- The 5-year survival following treatment with a well differentiated adenocarcinoma is approximately 75% for stage I, 55% for stage II, 35% for stage III and 10% for stage IV. The prognosis is worse with poorly differentiated tumours.

Box 20.6 Clinical staging of carcinoma of endometrium

Stage I	confined to corpus	*Ia*	length of uterine cavity less than 8 cm
		Ib	cavity longer than 8 cm
Stage II	involves corpus and cervix		
Stage III	extends outside uterus but not outside pelvis		
Stage IV	extends outside pelvis and/or involves bladder or rectal mucosa		

Management

- Full general and vaginal examination.
- Depends on fitness of patient and stage of the disease.
- If considered operable, treatment is by total hysterectomy and bilateral salpingo-oophorectomy with removal of a cuff of vagina. Lymph node involvement is looked for and para-aortic and pelvic nodes are sampled if enlarged.
- Preoperative intracavitary radiotherapy is given 6 weeks before surgery in some cases, e.g. stage II disease.
- Postoperative radiotherapy is given if the tumour is poorly differentiated, if there is penetration of more than the inner third of the myometrium by tumour or if the lymph nodes are involved. Treatment is with external radiotherapy to the pelvic walls, sometimes preceded by vaginal vault caesium.
- If the patient is unfit for surgery or the tumour is too advanced treatment is with radiotherapy.
- Progestogen treatment is indicated for residual tumour or recurrences – medroxy-progesterone acetate 100 mg twice or three times daily.
- Cytotoxic chemotherapy is not usually beneficial.
- Regular follow-up should be performed. Recurrences may occur in the vagina, in the pelvis or as distant metastases in the lungs or bone. Treatment is with a progestogen ± radiotherapy.

Sarcomas of the uterus

Presentation

- Usually present with abnormal bleeding.
- May present with pelvic pressure symptoms due to a mass.
- May present with generalized symptoms due to metastases.

Incidence

- Rare (account for less than 1% of genital tract cancers) but are often very malignant.

Aetiology

- Unknown.

Histology and pathology

- There are several types of sarcoma including leisomyosarcomas (arising in a fibroid or in the myometrium) and various forms of endometrial sarcoma.
- Spread is by local invasion and via lymphatics and the bloodstream.
- Overall 5-year survival is less than 35%.

Management

- An endometrial sarcoma may be diagnosed at curettage but a leiomyosarcoma is not usually diagnosed until histological examination following hysterectomy (or occasionally myomectomy) has been performed.
- Treatment is primarily surgical with total abdominal hysterectomy and bilateral salpingo-oophorectomy. Radiotherapy and chemotherapy are of limited value.
- Regular follow-up visits must be arranged.

Carcinoma of the fallopian tube

Presentation

- Patient usually in 40- to 60-year-old age group.
- Approximately 50% of patients are nulliparous.
- Seldom diagnosed prior to laparotomy.
- May present with vaginal bleeding or watery discharge (approximately 50%), pain (30%) or a mass (10%).

Incidence

Primary carcinoma of the tube is rare (less than 0.3% of cases of genital tract cancer). Secondary spread (usually from the ovary) is more common.

Histology and pathology

- Papillary adenocarcinoma.
- Purple swelling usually in the lateral part of the tube. Bilateral in 20% of cases.
- Five-year survival varies from 60% for early disease to 15% for late disease.

Management

- Treatment is surgical by total abdominal hysterectomy and bilateral salpingo-oophorectomy.
- Chemotherapy can be useful but radiotherapy is not of proven value.

Carcinoma of the ovary

Presentation

- Usually in 40- to 70-year-old age group but particularly the non-epithelial tumours can occur in younger women.
- Frequently asymptomatic until stage III or IV.
- May be found on a routine examination.
- Commonly presents with increase in girth and pressure symptoms related to the

size of the tumour and to the presence of ascites or with nausea, dyspepsia, weight loss and cachexia which may be due to small bowel obstruction.

- May rarely present with a complication such as torsion or rupture.
- Hormone-secreting tumours may present with endocrine effects such as amenorrhoea, hirsutism and postmenopausal bleeding.
- Findings on examination will depend on the stage of the disease. The tumour may or may not be palpable abdominally. There is often irregularity in the pouch of Douglas. Ascites is commonly present.

Incidence

- Approximately 4500 new cases in England and Wales per year.
- Approximately 3500 deaths in England and Wales per year.
- Accounts for approximately 50% of deaths from genital cancer.

Aetiology

- Uncertain.
- Commonest in industrialized societies and particularly in the Western World.
- Seems to be less common in women of high parity.
- A family history may be present.

Histology and pathology

- Ninety per cent of malignant ovarian tumours are of epithelial origin, most commonly serous and mucinous cystadenocarcinomas and endometrioid carcinomas.
- The remaining 10% includes those developing in ovarian stroma and sex cord and germ cell tumours and metastases from elsewhere.
- Spread is initially intraperitoneal. The omentum is frequently involved (Box 20.7).
- Metastatic tumours in the ovary are common and come mainly from the gastrointestinal tract, breast and endometrium.
- The 5-year survival following treatment is approximately 70% for stage Ia, 50% for stage IIa, 10% for stage III and less than 5% for stage IV. Overall 5-year survival is less than 25%.

Management

- Full general and vaginal examination.
- Ultrasound and magnetic resonance imaging cannot distinguish for certain between a benign and a malignant tumour (Figure 20.1).
- Laparotomy is required for diagnosis, staging and treatment.
- Peritoneal fluid is sent for cytology and an accurate description of the findings is

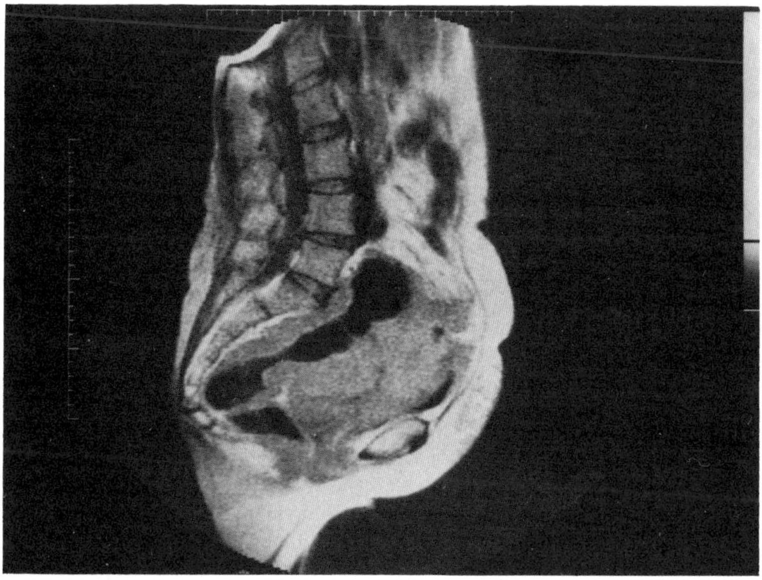

Figure 20.1 Magnetic resonance imaging of advanced primary ovarian cancer encircling rectum (TR 500 ms, TE 40 ms). (Courtesy of Mr Martin Powell).

Box 20.7 Staging of ovarian carcinoma

Stage I	limited to ovaries	*Ia*	limited to one ovary; no ascites (i) intact capsule; no tumour on surface (ii) ruptured capsule and/or tumour on surface
		Ib	limited to both ovaries; no ascites (i) intact capsules, no tumour on surface (ii) ruptured capsule(s) and/or tumour on surface
		Ic	Ia or Ib with ascites or positive peritoneal washings
Stage II	involves one or both ovaries with pelvic extension	*IIa*	involves uterus and/or tubes
		IIb	involves other pelvic organs
		IIc	IIa or IIb with ascites or positive peritoneal washings
Stage III	involves one or both ovaries with intraperitoneal metastases and/or retroperitoneal lymph nodes		
Stage IV	one or both ovaries with hepatic or distant metastases		

made with careful inspection of the liver, diaphragm, omentum, peritoneal surfaces, bowel and pelvis. The para-aortic nodes are palpated and removed if enlarged.

- Total hysterectomy, bilateral salpingo-oophorectomy and omentectomy are normally performed, with removal of any visible metastatic tumour (debulking procedure) in order to improve the efficacy of adjuvant therapy.
- In a young woman with stage Ia disease, radical treatment may be inappropriate and it is *essential* to be sure that the condition is malignant before embarking on radical surgery. Occasionally a serous cystadenoma may have papilliferous projections on the outer surface and in these cases ascites is commonly present. With stage Ia carcinoma in a young woman wishing to conserve her fertility, treatment is by unilateral oophorectomy.
- Adjuvant therapy includes chemotherapy and, rarely, radiotherapy.
- Platinum-based chemotherapy is frequently given. A variety of regimens have been used usually with treatment at monthly intervals for 6–12 months followed by second-look laparoscopy or laparotomy. Chemotherapy carries a considerable morbidity and should only be undertaken in a specialized unit.
- Regular follow-up is essential and will include history, general and vaginal examination with further investigations such as ultrasound as indicated.

Chapter 21

Uterovaginal displacement

The transverse cervical (cardinal) and uterosacral ligaments inserted into the upper parts of the cervix and of the vagina support the uterus and vault of the vagina in their normal situation in the pelvis. The round ligaments help to maintain the uterus in anteversion but, in about 15% of otherwise normal women, the uterus is retroverted.

Uterine displacement

The uterus may be displaced forwards or backwards, sideways, upwards or downwards.

Forward and upward displacement of the uterus

This may be due to previous surgery such as shortening of the round ligaments (ventrosuspension) or to the presence of a tumour or collection in the pouch of Douglas.

Lateral displacement of the uterus

This may be due to adhesions pulling the uterus sideways, or to a cyst or tumour pushing it sideways or to a congenital abnormality of the uterus such as a unicornuate or bicornuate uterus.

Backward displacement of the uterus

Retroversion of the uterus may be idiopathic (in approximately 15% of women) or due to adhesions – fixed retroversion – in endometriosis or chronic pelvic sepsis.

Downward displacement of the uterus

Prolapse of the uterus down the vagina is due to weakening of the supporting fascia and levator ani muscles.

Retroversion of the uterus

Diagnosis

- The cervix points forwards and may be up behind the symphysis pubis on vaginal examination. The body of the uterus is felt in the pouch of Douglas.
- It may not be easy to assess the size of the uterine body accurately unless (with a mobile retroversion) the cervix is pushed backwards and the uterine body is brought forwards using both the examining fingers and the abdominal palpating hand.

Types of retroversion

- *Mobile retroversion of the uterus* occurs in about 15% of normal women and is usually asymptomatic but is occasionally associated with deep dyspareunia. No treatment is usually required but if deep dyspareunia is thought to be related to the retroverted uterus and associated prolapse of the ovaries into the pouch of Douglas, the uterus can be anteverted and a Hodge pessary (Figure 21.1) inserted. If the symptoms are resolved the pessary is removed after 2 or 3 months and, if the symptoms return, it can be assumed that they were related to the retroverted uterus. Surgical maintenance of anteversion of the uterus (ventrosuspension) can then be considered.

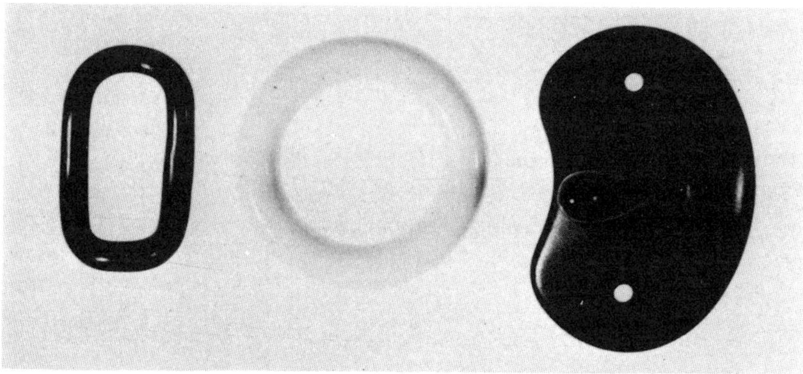

Figure 21.1 Hodge pessary, ring pessary and shelf pessary.

- *Fixed retroversion of the uterus* is usually due to adhesions in the pouch of Douglas either from chronic pelvic sepsis or endometriosis but may be due to impaction of a fibroid uterus. The symptoms will be related to the cause and usually include deep dyspareunia. Laparoscopy may be required to make a diagnosis. Treatment is the treatment of the cause.
- *Impacted retroverted gravid uterus* – a pregnant retroverted uterus will nearly always antevert spontaneously but occasionally this does not occur and it becomes impacted in the pelvis at about 14–16 weeks' gestation. The woman will usually present with urinary symptoms such as retention or retention with overflow. An indwelling urethral Foley catheter should be inserted into the bladder and left on free drainage; the patient must lie on her stomach and the uterus will nearly always come forward spontaneously.

Prolapse of the uterus

Uterine prolapse is associated with weakness of the supporting tissues which may be hereditary (and may occur in a nulliparous woman) or may be due to obstetric trauma. It becomes commoner after the menopause. The prolapse may be accentuated by increased intra-abdominal pressure due to a chronic cough or straining, or by obesity or occasionally an intra-abdominal tumour or ascites.

- *First degree prolapse* – slight descent of the axial or retroverted uterus. The cervix remains within the vagina.
- *Second degree prolapse* – the cervix appears at or protrudes through the introitus spontaneously or on straining.
- *Third degree prolapse* – complete procidentia. The entire uterus prolapses through the introitus. Ulceration (decubitus ulcer) of the cervix may occur – this heals readily if the prolapse is replaced in the vagina and held inside with an appropriate pessary. Oestrogen cream facilitates healing.
- *Symptoms and management* of uterine prolapse are discussed below.

Vaginal prolapse

This is often associated with uterine prolapse but each form of vaginal prolapse may occur on its own.

- *A urethrocele* is a prolapse of the lower third of the anterior vaginal wall and adjacent urethra.
- *A cystocele* is a prolapse of the upper two-thirds of the anterior wall and the adjacent bladder due to laxity of the pubocervical fascia. If the bladder base descends below the internal urethral meatus, there may be incomplete emptying of the bladder.
- *An enterocele* is a hernia of the pouch of Douglas through the posterior fornix of the vagina.
- *A rectocele* is a prolapse of the lower posterior wall of the vagina and rectum. There is often some associated deficiency of the perineal body.
- *Vault prolapse* is a term used to describe descent of the vaginal vault after abdominal or vaginal hysterectomy.

Symptoms caused by prolapse

- The presenting complaint is usually of something protruding through the introitus – 'a lump down below'.
- There may be urinary symptoms such as stress incontinence which may or may not be associated with a cystocele.
- A rectocele seldom causes difficulty with defaecation.
- When the cervix protrudes through the introitus it may become ulcerated and cause a blood-stained discharge.
- Backache is not usually caused by prolapse and it is important to explain this to the patient. If sacral backache is due to prolapse, it will be present on standing and will disappear on lying down.

History

- A general, obstetric and gynaecological history must be obtained seeking particularly for aetiological factors, associated and unassociated symptoms and possible contraindications to surgery.

- A careful history must be taken of any urinary symptoms.

Examination

- General examination, including blood pressure estimation, to exclude significant abnormalities and to assess fitness for surgery.
- Vaginal examination – speculum and bimanual examination followed by examination with Sims speculum in Sims (modified left lateral) position.

Investigations

- Cervical smear if appropriate.
- Microscopy and culture of the urine if indicated.
- If there are associated urinary symptoms such as urge incontinence urodynamic studies may be required (see Chapter 22).

Management

- Assess whether treatment is indicated and if so whether this should be conservative or surgical (Box 21.1). This will depend on the symptoms, the degree of prolapse, the wishes of the patient and whether she intends to have a pregnancy in the future and her fitness for surgery.

Box 21.1 Indications for conservative or no treatment in a woman with a prolapse

- Minimal symptoms or signs
- Does not want surgery
- Intends to have a pregnancy in the future
- Unfit for surgery
- While waiting for surgery

Conservative treatment for prolapse

- *Pelvic floor exercises* may be helpful if symptoms and signs are minimal. The aim is to improve the tone of the muscles of the pelvic floor. The patient is instructed to contract the muscles which are used voluntarily to stop micturition or defaecation.
- *A ring pessary* (Figure 21.1) is the most commonly used pessary. The correct size is determined using the index and middle fingers. It lies behind the symphysis pubis round the cervix with its posterior part in the posterior fornix. See Box 21.2 for details of insertion.
- *A shelf pessary* (Figure 21.1) should be used when surgery is contraindicated and the

tissues cannot hold a ring pessary, or the cervix and uterus prolapse through the ring. Intercourse is impossible if a shelf pessary is fitted.

Box 21.2 Insertion of a ring pessary

- Explain the purpose of the pessary and the method of insertion to the patient and show her the pessary
- Explain that once it is inserted she should not be aware of it and that it will not interfere with micturition, defaecation or intercourse
- Use the index and middle fingers to gauge the size of pessary required by assessing the distance from the symphysis pubis to the top of the posterior fornix
- Select the one which will fit well without exerting undue pressure on the vaginal walls
- Soften the pessary using hot water
- Squash the pessary to an elliptical shape to allow easy insertion and insert in the anteroposterior diameter of the introitus; once more than half the pessary is inserted allow it to turn through 90° and to come to lie in the correct position
- Check that it is inserted correctly and that the size is appropriate
- Ask the patient to walk about to determine whether she is aware of the pessary
- Explain to her how to remove the pessary if it becomes uncomfortable and that she need not worry if it falls out spontaneously
- Arrange to review in 6–8 weeks and then advise her to have the ring changed every 4–6 months and to present sooner if she has any discharge or bleeding
- When she comes to have the ring changed, remove the ring, inspect the vagina and cervix and perform a bimanual examination
- If there is any vaginal ulceration vaginal oestrogen cream should be prescribed; the ring may have to be left out for 2 or 3 weeks

Surgical treatment of prolapse

The operation required will depend on the symptoms and signs:

- *Anterior repair* (*colporrhaphy*) is used to treat a cystocele and/or urethrocele. Redundant vaginal wall is excised using a diamond-shaped or triangular incision, the bladder and urethra are pushed up after dissection, the pubocervical fascia is plicated and the vaginal wall is closed. A suprapubic or urethral catheter is often inserted at the time of operation to allow bladder drainage until micturition is re-established.

- *Posterior repair* (*colpoperineorrhaphy*) is used to treat a rectocele or enterocele. A triangular piece of vaginal wall is excised and the rectum is pushed back after dissection. If an enterocele is present the pouch of Douglas is opened, the neck of the sac is ligated and the redundant peritoneum is excised before approximating the uterosacral ligaments. The levator ani muscles are then approximated and the vaginal skin is closed. The perineal body is repaired if necessary.

Manchester repair

This is used in the treatment of uterovaginal prolapse when conservation of the uterus is desired. It consists of anterior colporrhaphy, amputation of the cervix, suturing of the divided cardinal ligaments in front of the cervix to antevert and to elevate the uterus, with posterior colpoperineorrhaphy if required.

- Amputation of the cervix should be avoided in women wanting further pregnancies.
- A posterior repair should only be performed if indicated and not as a routine. Dyspareunia is a common complication.

Vaginal hysterectomy and repair

This is performed when there is an indication for hysterectomy and for repair, and as the preferred treatment of prolapse by some surgeons when there is no contraindication to hysterectomy. There is a greater morbidity with this operation than with a Manchester repair. Vaginal hysterectomy is not appropriate when the uterus is enlarged to more than 12 weeks' size, or there is no descent of the uterus, or there are pelvic adhesions or when an anterior repair would be sufficient to treat the patient's symptoms.

Box 21.3 Preoperative management before repair operation or vaginal hysterectomy

- Assess fitness for surgery and treat significant medical problems (e.g. hypertension) appropriately
- Perform bladder studies if necessary
- Encourage weight loss if patient obese and cessation of smoking if she smokes
- Treat any vaginal or urinary infection that is present
- Give course of vaginal oestrogen cream if vagina is atrophic
- If there is cervical ulceration due to the prolapse treat it by replacing the cervix and retaining it in the vagina with a pessary and prescribe vaginal oestrogen cream

Box 21.4 Postoperative management after repair operation

- General care as for any major operation
- Prophylactic antibiotics are prescribed by some gynaecologists
- If a vaginal pack is inserted at operation this should be removed the next day
- Management of a suprapubic catheter varies from one gynaecologist to another. With a suprapubic catheter a period of drainage is usually followed by intermittent clamping and allowing the patient to micturate if she can. The residual (postmicturition) urine volume on 5 minutes free drainage should be less than 100 ml before the catheter is removed. A catheter specimen should be sent for microscopy and culture before the catheter is removed
- A vaginal examination should be performed before the patient goes home, if both anterior and posterior repairs were performed, to break down any adhesions

Complications of repair operations

- Those of any major operation, e.g. anaesthetic complications, deep vein thrombosis and pulmonary embolism.

- Reactionary and secondary haemorrhage. If bleeding is more than slight, it is usually wise to take the patient back to theatre for resuturing, or adequate insertion of a pack if bleeding points are not identified.
- Dyspareunia.
- Stress incontinence may occur even if it was not present preoperatively and may necessitate further surgery.
- Recurrence of prolapse may occur due to poor technique, failure to recognize and treat an enterocele or poor tissues. Transabdominal repair may be required. Colpocleisis is seldom performed.

Uterine inversion

This is an uncommon problem in which the fundus of the uterus is inverted and may protrude through the cervix. There are various degrees of inversion (Figure 21.2). An acute inversion is an obstetric complication of the third stage of labour requiring immediate replacement, whereas a chronic inversion may present as an obstetric (postpartum) or a gynaecological problem.

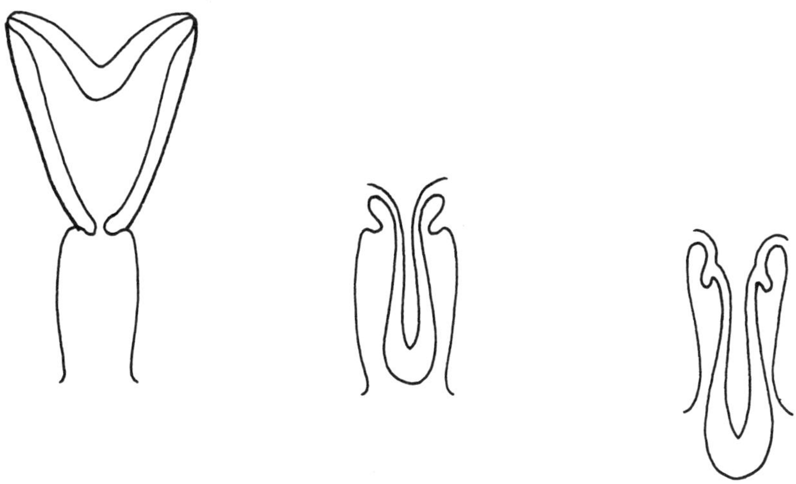

Figure 21.2 Inversion of uterus.

Aetiology of chronic uterine inversion

- Post partum – following unrecognized partial inversion of the uterus.
- Associated with a fibroid polyp which is extruded through the cervix and in doing so inverts the fundus of the uterus.

Presentation

- Discharge.

- Irregular (and sometimes extremely heavy bleeding with a fibroid polyp).
- Lower abdominal discomfort and intermittent labour-like pains.

Examination

- On vaginal examination there is often an ulcerated mass. The differential diagnosis is a carcinoma of the cervix, a fibroid polyp, a sarcoma or a uterine inversion.
- Examination under anaesthesia may be necessary to establish the diagnosis.

Management

- If a fibroid polyp presents through the cervix without inverting the uterus, it can be twisted off or the stalk can be transfixed and ligated.
- Chronic uterine inversion is difficult to reduce but this may be possible with a cup and stem pessary. If childbearing is completed hysterectomy may be a better option.

Chapter 22

Urinary incontinence and retention

Women complaining of urge or stress incontinence are traditionally referred to a gynaecologist.

It is important to distinguish between the various causes of incontinence.

Causes of urinary incontinence in a woman

- *Detrusor instability* or irritable bladder – normally presents with urge incontinence.
- *Sphincter weakness* – normally presents with stress incontinence.
- *Retention with overflow* – often due to neurological problem.
- *Congenital abnormalities and fistulae* – there is a continuous leak of urine.

Detrusor instability

Parasympathetic nerves (S2,3,4) sense distension and initiate bladder contractions which can be overcome by sympathetic stimulation (T11–L3) or voluntarily.

Detrusor instability may be due to one of a number of causes. Most commonly it is idiopathic but exacerbated by emotional stress, insecurity and anxiety.

Other causes include:

- Ovarian failure with lowered oestrogen levels.
- Inflammation of the urinary tract associated with infection, calculi or neoplasia.
- Neurological lesions such as multiple sclerosis.

Presentation

- If the bladder is not emptied immediately the desire to void is felt, there will be leakage of urine – urge incontinence. The woman complains that she has to 'go in a hurry'.
- Diurnal frequency is commonly complained of.
- Nocturnal frequency is less common but enuresis occasionally occurs especially in the young.
- An urge to micturate is precipitated by movement, by an increase in intra-abdominal pressure and by rapid filling of the bladder particularly following alcohol intake.
- The patient may be unduly anxious and may have a history of psychological problems or psychosomatic complaints.

Diagnosis

- The history is usually diagnostic. The combination of urge incontinence and frequency is very suggestive of bladder instability, but a urinary infection must always be excluded.
- Precipitating causes must be sought and a full general examination, including a neurological examination, must be carried out as well as a pelvic examination.
- A midstream urine specimen must be sent for microscopy and culture.
- Cystoscopy is occasionally indicated – if, for example, the woman also complains of haematuria.
- Cystometry (Figure 22.1 and Box 22.1) will demonstrate the diagnostic pattern of detrusor contractions during normal bladder filling.

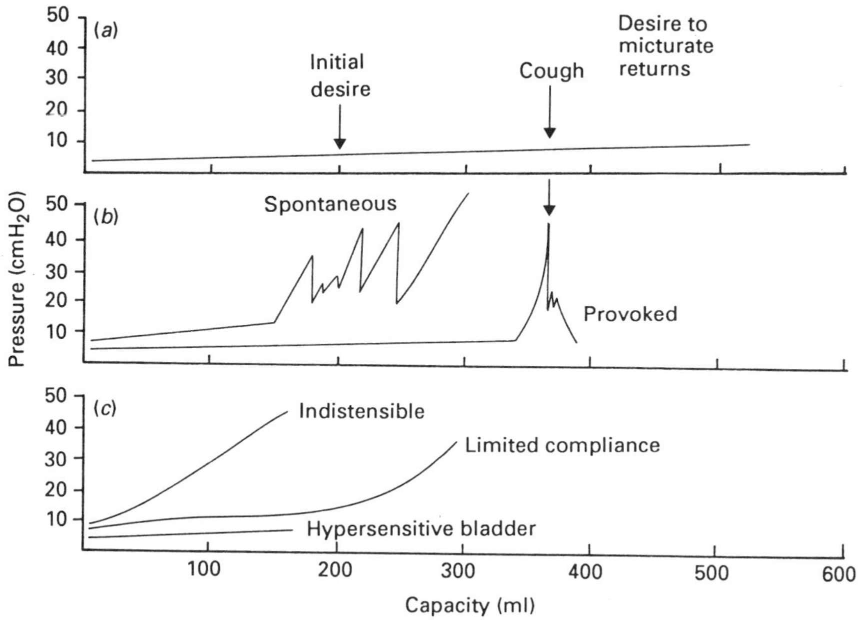

Figure 22.1 Cystometry: micturition occurs where the lines end. (*a*) Normal; (*b*) detrusor instability; (*c*) as indicated.

- Other studies such as micturating cystourethrography may be indicated when the diagnosis is unclear.

Management

- Treat any identified precipitating causes, e.g. urinary infection or oestrogen deficiency.
- Identify any underlying psychological problems and help the patient to have insight into their importance as a cause of the symptoms.
- *Bladder training* – patients are instructed to empty their bladder every hour by the

Box 22.1 Cystometry

- Urodynamic investigation designed to assess bladder detrusor function
- Appropriately zeroed pressure transducers are inserted into the bladder and rectum; the rectal transducer measures intra-abdominal pressure; subtraction of rectal pressure from intravesical pressure gives a measure of detrusor activity
- A physiological fluid such as physiological saline, at body temperature, is infused at approximately 50 ml per minute through a urethral catheter
- Normally a desire to micturate will be felt after 100–250 ml has been instilled; this desire can usually be overcome and will be felt again after 400–500 ml has been instilled
- Normal bladder capacity is 500–550 ml; a capacity over 800 ml is suggestive of defective bladder contractions
- The intravesical pressure (usually < 10 cmH_2O) should hardly change during bladder filling until capacity is reached if bladder compliance is normal
- A rise in intravesical pressure above 15 cmH_2O during filling or on provocation such as coughing suggests detrusor instability (Figure 22.1)

Indications for cystometry

- History of urge incontinence
- History of stress and urge incontinence
- Unexplained frequency
- Possible neurogenic bladder dysfunction
- Persistent stress and/or urge incontinence after surgery for incontinence

clock. The time interval is increased over a period of days or weeks to $1\frac{1}{2}$, 2, $2\frac{1}{2}$ and 3 hours. The aim is to break the habit of frequent micturition and to re-educate the bladder to tolerate larger volumes of urine. If the patient is well motivated the success rate is more than 80%.

- *Anticholinergic drugs* may be helpful if bladder training fails. Propantheline bromide 15 mg four times a day can be given with a success rate of approximately 60%. Side-effects include dry mouth, flushing and constipation. Contraindications include glaucoma and cardiac insufficiency.
- *β*-Sympathomimetic drugs can enhance the inhibitory effect of the sympathetic nervous system – salbutamol (Ventolin) and terbutaline sulphate (Bricanyl) can be tried.
- Other drugs which are sometimes helpful include calcium antagonists and antiprostaglandins.
- Antidepressants such as imipramine hydrochloride (Tofranil) and amitriptyline hydrochloride (Tryptizol) are often prescribed.

Urge and stress incontinence

When the patient presents with both urge and stress incontinence bladder studies are essential to determine the exact nature of the problem.

Box 22.2 Enuresis

Aetiology

- Normal in a young child until bladder control is learnt
- Can persist usually due to psychological problems
- May be due to the same underlying problems as urge incontinence

Management

- Exclude organic cause; if necessary perform bladder studies
- If no organic cause look for possible psychological problems
- Reduce fluid intake in the evening
- Anticholinergic or antidepressant drug may be helpful
- If persists try bladder training by getting the patient either to wake at intervals with an alarm clock in order to micturate, or to use electric bed buzzer
- Psychiatric referral is occasionally indicated

Box 22.3 Urethral syndrome

Characterized by recurrent attacks of frequency and dysuria without obvious pathology. It is associated with:

- Poor hygiene
- Contact allergy
- Oestrogen withdrawal
- Psychosexual or psychosocial problems

Management – exclude all possible underlying causes

Treatment – this can be very difficult in the absence of an identifiable cause

Sphincter weakness

Usually presents with stress incontinence.

- Occasional stress incontinence is normal on coughing or laughing.
- Recurrent stress incontinence is due to functional weakness of the internal urethral sphincter.
- The pubococcygeus muscle normally supports the bladder neck and maintains the posterior urethrovesical angle which should be approximately 1 cm behind and 1 cm above the lower edge of the symphysis pubis and less than 120° at rest.
- Damage to the bladder neck supports results in descent of the bladder neck below the intra-abdominal cavity, an increase in the posterior urethrovesical angle, funnelling of the upper urethra and stress incontinence.
- Stress incontinence will be aggravated by an increase in intra-abdominal pressure due to a chronic cough, obesity, pregnancy, intra-abdominal tumours and ascites.

It may also become worse postmenopausally because of a decrease in oestrogen levels.

Presentation

- The patient is normally a parous woman over 35 years of age, often with a history of a long labour and/or an assisted vaginal delivery.
- She will complain that she leaks a small amount of urine when she coughs, laughs or sneezes, even if the bladder is not particularly full. Voluntary contraction of the external sphincter prevents loss of a large quantity of urine.

Diagnosis

- A complete history is taken.
- General and abdominal examination precede vaginal examination.
- A routine vaginal examination is performed with speculum examination of the cervix and a bimanual examination. Stress incontinence may be demonstrated on coughing.
- The patient is then examined for prolapse in the left lateral position with a Sims speculum (see Chapter 1). Prolapse is not always present.

Investigations

- A midstream urine sample should be sent for culture and microscopy. Other investigations are not usually necessary if the history and examination are typical of stress incontinence.
- Cystometry and a micturating cystogram may be required if the history and findings are not clear-cut.

Treatment

The aim is to strengthen the support of the bladder neck and to elevate it into an intra-abdominal position and to restore the normal posterior urethrovesical angle. Treatment may be conservative or surgical.

- *Pelvic floor exercises* may be helpful in a young woman with minimal or no prolapse or in the postpartum period.
- *A ring pessary* (see Chapter 21) may be helpful as a temporary measure during pregnancy or in someone who does not wish to undergo, or who is not fit for, surgery, but is often of no help at all for stress incontinence. A reversed Hodge pessary may be more helpful.
- *Surgical treatment* (Figure 22.2) can be either by a vaginal or an abdominal or a combined approach.
  (1) *A vaginal approach* is often appropriate particularly when vaginal prolapse is also present. Following dissection the pubocervical fascia is plicated under the bladder neck to elevate and to support it and to restore the posterior urethrovesical angle. This approach is successful in approximately 80% of cases.

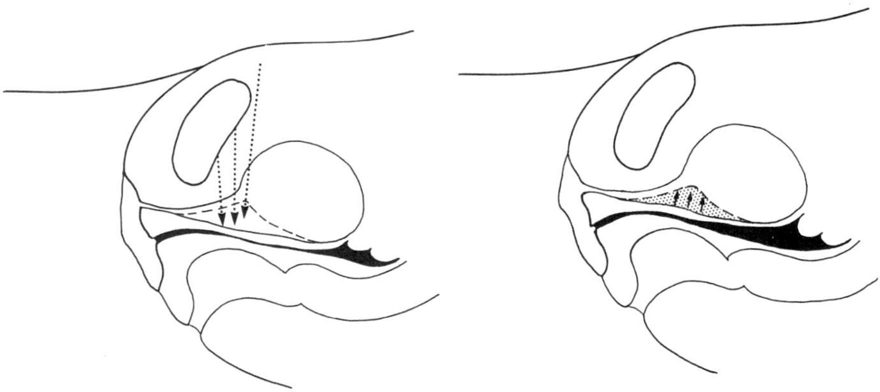

Figure 22.2 Surgery for stress incontinence. (*a*) Principle of abdominal approach; (*b*) principle of vaginal approach.

(2) *An abdominal approach* is increasingly preferred. The aim is to elevate the proximal urethra and bladder neck and to recreate the normal posterior urethrovesical angle using either synthetic or natural material. The vaginal or paraurethral tissues are anchored to the posterior aspect of the symphysis, to the pelvic brim or to the rectus sheath.
(3) In the Marshall–Marchetti–Krantz technique the para-urethral fascia is attached to the periosteum of the symphysis pubis, using a low transverse abdominal incision to gain access to the cave of Retzius.
(4) In the Burch procedure the vagina alongside the urethrovesical junction is attached to the ileopectineal ligament.
(5) In Stamey's procedure non-absorbable sutures are used to elevate the bladder neck and are stitched to the rectus sheath. A urethral sling can be made from fascia from the rectus sheath, animal fascia or synthetic material. It is threaded under the urethrovesical angle and attached to the recti.

- Success rate following primary surgery should be at least 90%. Failure may be due to inadequate preoperative assessment (Box 22.4) or poor technique or failure of patient to avoid straining postoperatively (Box 22.5).
- Delivery after successful surgery should be by caesarean section.

Box 22.4 Preoperative assessment

- Determine with patient whether treatment is indicated
- Perform cystometry if necessary
- Assess fitness for surgery
- Explain the procedure that will be performed and any likely consequences

Box 22.5 Postoperative management

- General care as for any major operation
- Suprapubic catheter usually left draining freely for 3–5 days – exact management differs from one surgeon to another
- Suprapubic catheter is clamped for 3 or 4 hours and patient is encouraged to attempt to pass urine. If patient unable to pass urine catheter is unclamped and urine drained, and then reclamped. Residual should be less than 100 ml before removing catheter
- Catheter specimen of urine collected for culture prior to removal of catheter
- Bowel contents must be kept soft and patient must avoid straining for 2–3 months

Retention and overflow incontinence

This is not a common problem in women. Possible non-obstetric causes include pelvic tumour, prolapse, neurological, postsurgery.

- Pelvic tumours which can cause retention of urine include haematocolpos, retroverted gravid uterus, ovarian tumour, pelvic haematocele and uterine fibroids (see Chapter 19).
- Occasionally a large cystocele may be associated with retention.
- Neurological causes include multiple sclerosis and neurological damage during radical pelvic surgery or when excessive overdistension of the bladder has been allowed to occur. Retention of urine may occur in geriatric patients.
- Retention of urine is common immediately following gynaecological surgery and traumatic childbirth and should be watched out for.
- Prolonged retention may follow repair operations and operations for stress incontinence and radical pelvic surgery.

Diagnosis

- History.
- Palpable symmetrical cystic mass arising from the pelvis.
- Catheterization will confirm the diagnosis.

Management

- Depends on the cause.
- Following surgery catheterization on one occasion is often all that is required. The patient will usually be able to pass urine once she is mobilized.

Congenital abnormalities and fistulae

Congenital abnormalities leading to retention or incontinence are usually dealt with in childhood. Occasionally, incontinence due to an aberrant ureter may not present until later.

Acquired fistulae

These may be caused by direct trauma (during surgery), avascular necrosis (during labour and delivery or in relation to an inappropriately inserted suture), malignancy – particularly carcinoma of the cervix or following radiotherapy.

Presentation

- There will usually be a history of a possible precipitating cause.
- With a vesicovaginal fistula there will be continuous leakage of urine and the patient will not need to empty the bladder.
- With a ureteric fistula there will be continuous leakage of urine but also intermittent emptying of the bladder following filling from the other ureter.

Diagnosis

- Methylene blue test.
- Intravenous urogram and cystoscopy will usually be indicated.

Treatment

- A small vesicovaginal fistula of recent origin should be treated by catheterization and continuous drainage for 3 weeks. Spontaneous healing may occur. If formal repair is required this should be performed with or by a urologist.
- The repair of a ureteric fistula should be undertaken by a urologist.

Chapter 23
Menopause

Menopause implies cessation of menstruation. Difficult to diagnose for certain except in retrospect. Six months amenorrhoea around the time of the menopause is arbitrarily taken to imply that the menopause has occurred.

- Average age of menopause in the West is 51 years (normal range 47–55 years).
- Average life expectancy at 50 is a further 30 years and, as life expectancy increases, the implications of long-term low oestrogen levels become more important.
- More than 75% of postmenopausal women have symptoms related to oestrogen deficiency at some time. In about 25% of women the symptoms are severe enough to interfere significantly with their daily life.
- There are advantages and disadvantages of oestrogen replacement therapy which have not been fully evaluated and a decision on whether or not to advise replacement therapy for a particular woman must be based on a detailed knowledge of her medical history and present circumstances.

Changes that occur are listed in Box 23.1 and common problems arising in Box 23.2.

Box 23.1 Changes that occur around and after the time of the menopause

Pituitary	increased production of FSH and LH
Skeletal	negative calcium balance
Blood	haematocrit↑ LDL↑ HDL↓ FSH↑, LH↑
Ovaries	decrease in size, few remaining follicles. Loss of cyclic oestrogen and progesterone production but continuation of androgen production which, with adrenal androgen production and peripheral conversion of androgens to oestrogens, gives average postmenopausal circulating oestradiol levels of 30–50 pmol/l
Uterus	↓ from 100–120 g to 50–60 g in weight and even less in older women. Endometrium thin and cuboidal but responds to oestrogen
Cervix	atrophies and canal narrows. Squamocolumnar junction moves up canal
Vagina	vaginal epithelium thins and glycogen production decreases leading to an increase in pH and to atrophic vaginitis
Bladder and urethra	epithelium thins and atrophic trigonitis and urethritis may ensue
Vulva	gradual atrophy, decreased hair

Hot flushes

- True hot flushes and sleep disturbance associated with hot flushes are definitely related to low oestrogen levels.

Box 23.2 Common problems that may arise around and after the time of the menopause, some of which are related to decreased oestrogen levels and others to ageing

Neuroendocine	hot flushes, sleep disturbance, psychological problems, decreased libido
Skeletal	backache, osteoporosis, fractures
Breasts	smaller and less firm
Skin	loss of pliability and resilience, atrophy, dry hair, decreased number of hair follicles and decrease of sweat and sebaceous gland activity, increased facial hirsutism
Cardiovascular	increased incidence of atheroma, hypertension and myocardial infarction. Decreased genital tract blood flow
Vagina	vaginal dryness, vaginitis, dyspareunia, blood-stained discharge, increasing incidence of prolapse
Bladder and urethra	dysuria, frequency and urgency, urge incontinence
Vulva	atrophy, pruritus vulvae

- Last for a few seconds to several minutes. Sudden onset of reddening of skin over head, neck and chest accompanied by feeling of heat and followed by sometimes profuse perspiration.
- May be precipitated by heat or anxiety.
- May persist for at least a year in the majority of those affected or for several years in a minority.
- Exact cause unclear but related to reduction in oestrogen levels which leads to alterations in brain catecholamine levels; this, in turn, affects the hypothalamic temperature regulating centre causing a decrease in the core temperature set point. This leads to peripheral vasodilatation and sweating and also a simultaneous release of LHRH and hence of LH.
- Oestrogen therapy is the best treatment for true hot flushes and for the sleep disturbance associated with them. There is also some effect with placebo treatment. Treatment with a progestogen can sometimes be beneficial when oestrogen therapy is contraindicated.

Psychological problems

These are often complex in origin and are related to changing social circumstances as well as to the menopause. They arise most commonly in those who have had previous problems. Explanation and reassurance may be all that is required in approximately half those women presenting with psychological problems around time of menopause.

Decreased libido

- This too may be related to changing social circumstances rather than to changing hormone levels.

- Hormone treatment with oestrogen and occasionally androgen (mainly in those who have had a bilateral oophorectomy) may sometimes be indicated.

Skeletal changes

- After the age of 40 bone density in women (and men to a lesser extent) begins to decrease.
- Trabecular bone is affected first with increased rate of vertebral and wrist fractures in 50- to 65-year-olds; then increasing cortical bone loss causes increased incidence of hip fractures in older age group.

Box 23.3 Risk factors for osteoporosis

- Increasing age
- Female sex
- Ethnic predisposition (commoner in White and Asian women than in Black women)
- Family history
- Low calcium intake throughout life
- Early menopause or oophorectomy
- Lack of exercise
- Nulliparity
- Cigarette smoking
- High intake of alcohol, sodium, caffeine, protein or phosphate
- Other causes of increased bone loss – corticosteroid treatment, Cushing's syndrome, hyperthyroidism, hyperparathyroidism, gastrointestinal or bone marrow disease

Role of oestrogen therapy in prevention of osteoporosis

- Mode of action of oestrogen on bone is still unclear (no oestrogen receptors have been found in bone). However, it definitely decreases urinary output of calcium and hydroxyproline; serum calcium, phosphorus and alkaline phosphatase levels fall on treatment with oestrogen.
- Prolonged oestrogen replacement therapy reduces bone loss and the incidence of fractures in later life to a level comparable with that in men of the same age.
- Progestogens can also help to reduce bone loss, calcium is less effective.
- No really satisfactory methods available for measurement of bone mass – all current methods have disadvantages; serial measurements are necessary to determine significance of results.

Cardiovascular system

- Definite increase in incidence of myocardial infarction after the menopause but at least partly age related.

- LDL raised and HDL decreased after the menopause. These changes can be reversed by oestrogen therapy but some of the beneficial effect of oestrogen is negated by progestogen therapy.
- Increasing clinical evidence of a probable reduction in incidence of myocardial infarction in women receiving oestrogen replacement therapy, especially those with premature ovarian failure.

Genital tract

- Oestrogen treatment has definite beneficial effects on genital tract blood flow and on vaginal epithelium and on symptoms due to atrophic changes in the lower genital and urinary tracts. Dyspareunia is also reduced if regular intercourse occurs.
- Long-term unopposed oestrogen treatment can also have adverse effects on the genital tract. There is a dose- and duration-dependent increase in the incidence of carcinoma of the endometrium with unopposed oestrogen and this increased risk continues after oestrogen therapy has been discontinued.
- The addition of an adequate dose of progestogen for 12 days every 4 weeks appears to reduce the incidence of atypical hyperplasia and endometrial adenocarcinoma dramatically. Progestogens reduce epithelial DNA synthesis and therefore antagonize the mitotic effects of oestrogen. Progestogens, however, also have unwanted side-effects and therefore the dose should be the minimum required for endometrial protection but unfortunately varies from person to person.
- At the present time adequate doses of progestogens for most women appear to be as follows: medroxyprogesterone acetate 10 mg once a day, norethindrone 0.7 mg once a day, norethisterone 5 mg once a day, norgestrel 150 μg once a day; it is not certain what constitutes an adequate dose of the other progestogens.
- If bleeding only occurs after the end of each progestogen course (usually 1–3 days later), it is likely that adequate change to secretory endometrium has occurred.
- Best method of follow-up of women on long-term hormone replacement therapy has not been determined but, provided adequate doses of progestogen are taken and the bleeding pattern is as above, they are probably adequately protected and only require curettage if abnormal bleeding occurs.
- Attempts have been made to produce an adequate and safe oestrogen and progestogen regimen which does not cause vaginal bleeding but the ideal combination has not yet been found.

Choice of oestrogen for hormone replacement therapy

- Conflicting evidence about superiority of different oestrogens.
- The various available oestrogens affect different systems and different women to a different degree and an effect on a particular system thus varies with the oestrogen given, with the dose and with the route of administration.

- Therefore not possible to give exactly equivalent potencies but orally 1 mg oestradiol valerate, 1 mg 17β-oestradiol and 5 μg ethinyl oestradiol are roughly equivalent to 0.625 mg conjugated oestrogen (Premarin) which is the average dose required for control of symptoms and for prophylaxis against osteoporosis.
- Oestrogen should be given either cyclically or continuously, with a progestogen for 12 days out of every 28 days.
- The theoretical advantage of oestrogen administration using implants and patches is that the metabolism in the gut wall and the 'first pass through the liver' effect is avoided and, therefore, there are less unwanted hepatic effects; however the long-term epidemiological benefits have not been fully evaluated. Cyclical progestogen therapy is still required to protect the endometrium.
- Debatable whether addition of a progestogen is required (to protect the breasts) in a woman who has had a hysterectomy and progestogens can have deleterious effects on lipid levels.
- If oestrogen therapy is contraindicated, progestogen therapy may alleviate hot flushes and gives some protection against the development of osteoporosis.

Management of patient requesting advice about hormone replacement therapy

History

- *Ask about symptoms* that could be due to oestrogen deficiency and about any other symptoms.
- *Menstrual history* to ensure no abnormal bleeding is occurring.
- *Assess psychosocial situation.*
- *Determine any possible contraindications* to oestrogen replacement therapy, such as breast cancer or other hormone-dependent neoplasia, previous thromboembolic disease, other vascular disease including significant hypertension, liver disease, fibroids, endometriosis.

Examination

- General examination including blood pressure and breast examination.
- Vaginal examination and cervical smear if indicated.

Investigations

Occasionally measurement of FSH and/or oestradiol levels may be indicated if uncertain whether symptoms are due to menopause.

Treatment

- Discussion of cause of any symptoms and of likely duration of symptoms such as hot flushes.
- Discussion of advantages (Box 23.4) and disadvantages (Box 23.5) of hormone replacement therapy.

Box 23.4 Advantages of oestrogen replacement therapy

- Alleviation of symptoms due to oestrogen deficiency
- Reduction in incidence of osteoporosis and of vertebral, wrist and hip fractures
- Possible reduction in incidence of myocardial infarction

Box 23.5 Disadvantages of oestrogen replacement therapy

- Increased incidence of endometrial hyperplasia and carcinoma if an adequate amount of progestogen is not taken
- Withdrawal bleeding which may be associated with dysmenorrhoea
- Breast tenderness
- Possible increased risk of thromboembolism

Choice of treatment

- Oral plus progestogen.
- Implant or transdermal plus progestogen.
- Vaginal plus progestogen (a short course of vaginal oestrogen therapy – such as dienoestrol cream may be given without added progestogen for local symptoms but it must be remembered that there is very good absorption of oestrogen from the vagina).

Duration of treatment

- Will depend on individual situation and should be kept under review.
- The woman should be seen every 6 months and asked about any abnormal symptoms. She should have a general examination including breast examination and blood pressure estimation.
- A vaginal examination should be performed annually or more often if indicated.

Further reading

Dewhurst C.J. (1984). Female puberty and its abnormalities. *Current Reviews in Obstetrics and Gynaecology 9.* Churchill Livingstone, London.

Guillebaud J. (1985). *Contraception – your questions answered.* Pitman Publishing, London.

Studd, J. (Ed.) (1981–1987). *Progress in Obstetrics and Gynaecology, Volumes 1–6.* Churchill Livingstone, London.

Whitfield, C.R. (Ed.) (1986). *Dewhurst's Textbook of Obstetrics and Gynaecology for Postgraduates,* 4th edn. Blackwell, London.

Wilson, E.A. (Ed.) (1987). *Endometriosis.* Alan R. Liss Inc., New York.

Index